This is a short, up-to-date book giving an account of the development of the nervous systems in both invertebrates and vertebrates. It describes the nervous system at all stages of development from the early embryo, when nerve cells first appear, through to the adult, when interaction between nerve cells is the basis of learning, memory and recovery from injury. The emphasis is on fundamental concepts and the book is intended for undergraduates and graduates and as a source book for those teaching courses in neuronal development. The large number of references will also make it useful to the researcher.

ESSENTIALS OF NEURAL DEVELOPMENT

ESSENTIALS OF NEURAL DEVELOPMENT

M.C. Brown
Lecturer, Department of Physiology, University of Oxford
Fellow and Tutor, Trinity College, Oxford

W.G. Hopkins
Senior Lecturer, Department of Physiology, University of Otago

and

R.J. Keynes
Lecturer, Department of Anatomy, University of Cambridge

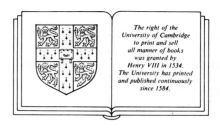

*The right of the
University of Cambridge
to print and sell
all manner of books
was granted by
Henry VIII in 1534.
The University has printed
and published continuously
since 1584.*

CAMBRIDGE UNIVERSITY PRESS
CAMBRIDGE
NEW YORK   PORT CHESTER
MELBOURNE   SYDNEY

Published by the Press Syndicate of the University of Cambridge
The Pitt Building, Trumpington Street, Cambridge CB2 1RP
40 West 20th Street, New York, NY 10011, USA
10 Stamford Road, Oakleigh, Melbourne 3166, Australia

First published 1984 as *Development of Nerve Cells and their Connections* by W.G. Hopkins and M.C. Brown and
© Cambridge University Press 1984

This revised edition published in 1991 as *Essentials of Neural Development* by M.C. Brown, W.G. Hopkins and R.J. Keynes and
© Cambridge University Press 1991

Printed in Great Britain at the University Press, Cambridge

British Library cataloguing in publication data

Brown, M. C. (Michael Charles)
Essentials of neural development.
1. Man. Nerves. Cells. Physiology
I. Title   II. Hopkins, W. G.   III. Keynes, R. J.   IV.
Hopkins, W. G. Development of nerve cells and their
connections
611.0181

Library of Congress cataloguing in publication data

Brown, M. C. (Michael Charles)
Essentials of neural development / M.C. Brown, W.G. Hopkins, and
R.J. Keynes.
    p. cm.
'A revised version of Development of nerve cells and their
connections by W.G. Hopkins & M.C. Brown.'
Includes bibliographical references.
Includes index.
ISBN 0-521-37556-8 (hardback). – ISBN 0-521-37698-X (paperback)
1. Developmental neurology. 2. Nerves. 3. Neurons. 4. Nerve
endings. I. Hopkins, W. G. II. Keynes, R. J. III. Hopkins, W. G.
Development of nerve cells and their connections. IV. Title.
[DNLM: 1. Neurons. WL 102.5 B879e]
QP363.5.H66   1991
591.1'88–dc   90-1975   CIP

ISBN 0 521 37556 8 hardback
ISBN 0 521 37698 X paperback

SE

Contents

Preface

This short book is intended to provide undergraduates and graduates with a simple framework of our present understanding of each stage of neuronal development, onto which new information can be readily grafted. Although only intended as an introductory text, we have included quite a large selection of references to original papers and reviews as these may prove useful to graduates and teachers, and to have left them out might have proved irritating. We have assumed that the readers already know at least some elementary neurophysiology, neurohistology, neuroanatomy and some general embryology.

The book is a revised and updated edition of our earlier book *Development of Nerve Cells and Their Connections* (by W.G.H. and M.C.B.).

Acknowledgements

We should like to thank Drs C.M. Booth, E.R. Lunn and V.H. Perry for critically reading early drafts of this book and providing useful suggestions. Drs E.R. Lunn and P. Jeffs drew most of the diagrams using Macdraw and we are very grateful to them for all the time and trouble they have taken.

Part 1

Introduction

Chapter 1

A short outline of neuronal development

Introduction

The nervous system is arguably the most complex structure known to man, and certainly the most complex organ system in the body. This is due in part to its large number of cells (about 10^{12} neurons in man and at least as many glial cells), and in part to its large variety of cell types (probably several hundreds or possibly even thousands). In both these respects other organ systems are comparable with the nervous system: for example, there are as many cells in the digestive system, and at least as many different kinds of cell in the immune system. But the nervous system differs from any other part of the body in that neurons make precise patterns of connections onto other neurons, so generating a remarkable diversity of structure and function.

Not surprisingly, many features of the development of the nervous system are still mysterious. In recent years an increasingly large number of scientists have become involved with research on developmental neurobiology, and it is probable that newly developed techniques will help solve many of the problems that have daunted previous generations of neurobiologists. Investigation of neuronal development, as is the case in most other fields, is carried out both because of the intrinsic curiosity of those concerned, and also because a better understanding of the mechanisms involved will benefit humanity. Abnormalities arising in development and as a result of disease or accident later in life may be alleviated by application of the new knowledge, and a better understanding of brain development will probably provide a better understanding of normal brain function.

In this introductory chapter there is a very brief outline of the normal sequence of events in brain development, then the methods and the design of experiments used in research in this field are given in Chapter 2.

Summary of the stages of neuronal development

In vertebrate embryos the cells whose descendants give rise to the nervous system are first identified as the neural ectoderm, a plate of cells in the midline of the early embryonic ectoderm. This rounds up to form a tube underneath the surface ectoderm. Further regional elongation, outpocketing, folding and thickening of this tube produces the gross anatomical

3

Table 1.1. *Stages in the growth of vertebrate nerve cells.*

Genesis of nerve cells	Proliferation, specification and migration
Establishing connections	{ Axon growth, dendritic growth { Synapse formation
Modifying connections	{ Nerve cell death { Reorganisation of initial inputs
Adult plasticity	{ Learning { Nerve growth after injury

divisions of the central nervous system. At the time of closure of the neural tube some cells break away to form a transient structure called the neural crest. The cells of the crest migrate away from the neural tube and form the ganglia and supporting cells of the peripheral nervous system. The fibre tracts and peripheral nerves are produced when nerve cells send out axons to their targets.

At the cellular level four major stages in brain development can be identified. These follow each other more or less consecutively and we have made these the basis for the four main subdivisions (Parts 2,3,4 and 5) of this book (see Table 1.1).

Part 2 (Genesis of nerve cells) is concerned with the origin of nerve cells. In vertebrates, commitment of embryonic cells to neuronal development has long been known to begin at the gastrula stage, when mesoderm, migrating under the ectoderm, induces it to become neural ectoderm. The neural ectoderm forms into the neural tube, which goes on to become the CNS. **Proliferation** of nerve cells occurs initially only along the inner surface of the neural tube, and later at a few sites on the outer surface of the brain. This is followed by **migration** of the postmitotic neurons radially through adjoining nerve tissue to their characteristic locations, guided by surface interactions with radially-oriented glial cell processes. In some parts of the CNS **specification of phenotypes**, the process whereby cells develop particular identities, has been shown to occur at the time of final mitosis. Cells of the peripheral nervous systems are derived from the neural crest, an aggregate of cells that detaches from the developing neural tube. The cells migrate out into the periphery along specific pathways with surfaces that are different from surrounding tissues. Specific phenotypes of the peripheral nervous system are induced by local influences.

In invertebrate species it has been possible to follow the development of specific, identified neurons from earlier precursor cells. These studies have revealed stereotyped patterns of cell division and cell differentiation, suggesting that the characteristics of particular neurons are determined at least partly by their ancestry or lineage. However, it appears that some neuronal phenotypes are also determined by an inductive process whereby uncommitted precursor cells develop their characteristics by interacting with their environment. In certain systems the inducing signals and their receptors are becoming known.

Part 3 (Establishing connections) deals with the ways neurons send their axons to establish connections with one another and with peripheral targets. Neurons elaborate an axon and usually also dendrites in order to make and receive connections. Growth of the axon and dendrites occurs at the advancing tips of these processes. These form a specialised structure called the **growth cone**, where material transported from the cell body is incorporated into both the cytoskeleton and membrane. The study of growth cones in tissue culture has shown that they need to attach to a surface in order to grow. They can be guided by differential adhesion to surfaces containing different molecules but also by weak electric fields and gradients of diffusible substances.

In the developing animal it has been found that **guidance of axons** occurs both by non-specific means along preformed pathways, and also by some 'active' mechanism that can direct axons arising from particular locations towards a particular target or even part of a target area. Further refinements in establishing specific connections can then occur by means of mutual **recognition** between the axons and their targets based upon some form of chemoaffinity.

Contact between axons and appropriate target cells results in **synaptogenesis**, which has been studied predominantly at the neuromuscular junction. Receptors for transmitter, having been distributed widely before innervation, become localised to the developing postsynaptic junctional membrane, while specialised release sites are induced in the presynaptic nerve terminal. Full maturation of the mammalian neuromuscular junction requires firing of action potentials by the postsynaptic cell. The peripheral branch of sensory axons takes part in the development of specialised sensory end-organs, but little is known about the mechanisms that underlie this. Interactions also occur between axons and their glial cells: in peripheral nerves contact with axons stimulates glial cells to divide, then to differentiate into the specialised glia of myelinated and unmyelinated nerves.

Part 4 (Modification of connections) discusses modifications that occur in the pattern of connections between nerve and target cells as synapses begin to form. The first of these modifications is **neuronal cell death**, which removes a variable but usually large proportion of the neurons that have sent out axons to their targets. Cell death probably eliminates errors in the initial pattern of connections and matches pre- and post-synaptic cell numbers. The mechanism underlying neuronal cell death is not fully understood, but it may depend upon electrical activity in the nerve–target pathways and involve uptake by the neurons of substances essential for their survival. One of the substances required for the survival of sympathetic neurons and dorsal root ganglion cells is a well-characterised protein called Nerve Growth Factor.

The second major modification of connections is the **elimination and reorganisation of terminal branches**, which occurs after the period of cell death. When axons reach their targets they branch and contact more postsynaptic cells than they do in the adult. These extra branches are also usually distributed more widely than in the adult. Some of the initial axonal branches are subsequently eliminated or redistributed. The mechanism for the elimination, like that for cell death, is dependent upon electrical activity, and a competition between the axon terminals for a factor (possibly the same as is involved in neuronal survival) may be involved.

During this stage of development it has been found that many neuronal connections are easily and permanently modified by alterations in the normal patterns of neural activity induced by environmental stimuli. This phenomenon has been studied extensively in the mammalian visual cortex, where it is found that abnormal visual experience produces abnormally responding neurons. The changes in the response properties of the neurons can be brought about most readily during a certain relatively short time interval, the so-called **critical period**. The neuroanatomical basis for critical periods is probably the presence of the excess and widespread presynaptic nerve branches, which provide an initial diffuse array of connections out of which the normal adult pattern can be sculpted. It appears that presynaptic inputs that release transmitter in close synchrony with postsynaptic cell firing are the ones which survive.

Part 5 (Adult plasticity) looks at changes that can occur in the mature nervous system. After the critical period, plasticity on a major scale is lost and neuronal connections become more permanent. However, plasticity in the adult in response to experience must also be present in neuronal pathways in order to account for **learning and memory**. Several convenient pathways in the adult mammalian CNS have been found where plasticity can be readily demonstrated and its biochemical and structural basis studied, notably in the hippocampus. Changes in transmission in pathways mediating a modifiable reflex response in the invertebrate *Aplysia* have also been studied in some detail.

Interactions between nerves and their target and glial cells continue to occur following the establishment of the relatively stable pattern of connections in the adult. The axon is the link between the nerve cell body and the other cells involved and transection of the axon interrupts the interactions and causes changes in nerve, target and glial cells. These interactions have been described as **trophic influences** (from the Greek *trophe*, food or sustenance) because they are necessary to maintain the cell properties associated with the innervated state. Trophic interactions occur in both the orthograde direction (the nerve cell maintaining its target and glial cells) and in the retrograde direction (the target and glial cells maintaining the nerve cell and its branches). Trophic interactions in the adult are important in relation to development of the nervous system in that they probably represent the continued operation of mechanisms that were in play during formation of the nervous system.

The final chapter of this section deals with changes in connections that occur following **injury** to the nervous system. These changes usually involve **regrowth** of damaged axons and **sprouting** of remaining intact axons and terminals in the vicinity of the degenerating nerves. Both forms of growth can reinnervate and restore function to denervated cells. The development of the new outgrowths appears to be controlled partly by the reversion of the denervated tissues to an embryonic state that can stimulate nerve growth and accept innervation, and also by the availability of suitable pathways for the sprouting or regenerating nerves to follow. Injury or suppression of activity in some pathways can also activate other pathways that are normally suppressed or undetectable.

Background reading

Alberts, B., Bray, D., Lewis, J., Raff, M., Roberts, K. & Watson, J.D. (1989). *Molecular Biology of the Cell.* 2nd edition. New York and London, Garland. Chapters 16 and 19.

Cowan, W.M. (1979). The development of the brain. *Scientific American*, **241** (September), 56–69.

Hamburger, V. (1981). Historical landmarks in neurogenesis. *Trends in Neuroscience*, **4**, 151–5.

Patterson, P. & Purves, D. (1982). *Readings in Developmental Neurobiology*, Cold Spring Harbor, Cold Spring Harbor Laboratory.

Purves, D. & Lichtman, J.W. (1985). *Principles of Neural Development.* Sunderland, MA, Sinauer.

Trends in Neuroscience, **8**, (1985). June. Special 'Fly and Worm' Issue.

Chapter 2

Methods and techniques

Anatomical methods

The greatest technical problem in developmental neurobiology has always been to make neurons visible. Indeed, the science began with Ramon y Cajal's use of a nerve-specific silver stain, which was discovered in the last century by Golgi and which is still widely used today. A short summary of methods used for identifying neurons and neuron processes in developmental studies is given below.

Silver stains. These are either of the Golgi type, which stain completely a small proportion of neurons, or of the reduced silver type, which stain all nerve processes with variable efficiency.

Electron microscopy has provided most of the knowledge about cellular structures important in cell migration, axon growth, synaptogenesis and remodelling of connections. Many of the methods devised for identifying particular neurons in the light microscope have been adapted to EM; but many questions still remain to be answered at the level of light microscopy.

Histochemistry. Some neurons can be visualised by means of their transmitter or transmitter enzymes. Catecholamines fluoresce in ultraviolet light in formaldehyde-fixed tissue and this has been very useful in assaying the presence of adrenergic neurons. Cholinergic neurons can be detected by the presence of accompanying acetylcholinesterase.

Horseradish peroxidase (HRP). This enzyme is transported within cells, both towards and away from the cell body. It can be injected or cells will take it up spontaneously. It is used to trace pathways or identify cell bodies when fixed sections of tissue are incubated with appropriate substrate. HRP is retained in the descendants of dividing cells and can be used to identify clones.

Fluorescent markers. These are visualised with ultraviolet microscopy. Some like HRP are transported within cells. Others, such as the carbocyanine dye DiI, are lipid-soluble and diffuse within the plane of the cell membrane. For lineage studies, clones can be labelled by iontophoresing non-toxic fluorescent markers (e.g. lysine–rhodamine–dextran) into single parent cells. The marker is too large to pass through gap junctions, and is therefore confined to the descendants of the cell.

Immunohistochemistry. Sera, or monoclonal antibodies specific for particular cell antigens, are bound to tissues and then revealed 'indirectly' by binding anti-antibodies coupled with HRP or fluorescent markers.

Autoradiographic tracing. Radioactive substances are transported along nerves and are visualised by autoradiography of sectioned material. In some cases the labelled material crosses synapses and delineates further pathways (trans-neuronal autoradiography).

Chimaeras. These are formed when embryonic neural cells (and their descendants) from one species are transplanted to another. The transplanted cells are identified subsequently in the chimaera through interspecies differences in histology of cells, e.g. structure of the nucleolus. Cells transplanted from an animal of the same species can be identified in a chimaera if they are prelabelled with an intracellular marker, for example HRP or fluorescent dye.

Birth-dating of neurons. A pulse of tritiated thymidine is incorporated into the DNA of the dividing precursors of nerve and glial cells and detected in these cells or their descendants by autoradiography. Dividing cells can also be labelled using a thymidine analogue, bromodeoxyuridine (BrdU), which is incorporated into cells undergoing DNA synthesis (S phase) and which can be visualised in histological sections using a monoclonal antibody against BrdU.

Recombinant retroviruses are used for tracing cell lineage. Retroviruses are made incapable of replication by replacing essential structural genes with a bacterial β-galactosidase gene. When the retrovirus infects a parent cell, its genome incorporates into the host genome and is inherited by the descendants of that cell; the β-galactosidase is expressed in all descendants, allowing the resultant clone to be identified histochemically. New virions are not produced, so neighbouring, unrelated cells are not labelled. This technique has been useful for examining cell lineage in brain areas that are difficult to label by intracellular injection with fluorescent markers or HRP.

Direct long term observation of neurons in vivo. The use of fluorescent vital dyes to stain nerve cells, in combination with low light level video microscopy and suitable image processing, has allowed the direct, repeated observation of individual cells and their processes *in vivo* over long time periods, for example several months.

Physiological methods

Patterns of central connections and changes in these patterns have been assayed by extracellular recording of action potentials from single cells or small clusters of cells, using wire or glass microelectrodes. Intracellular recording has been used to detect development of innervation and the changes in inputs to individual cells in the peripheral and central nervous system. Connections can also be determined by detecting biochemical changes arising from activity in particular axons or pathways. Functional changes in developing ion channels can be detected by the method of patch clamping. In muscle, the fibres comprising a single motor unit can be identified histochemically if their glycogen levels are depleted by prior activation. For neurons a non-metabolisable glucose analogue (2-deoxyglucose) can accumulate in active cells and its presence can be detected autoradiographically.

Biochemical and molecular biological methods

Levels of transmitter and transmitter enzymes in some tissues have been used to determine changes in innervation. Effects of innervation or denervation on transmitter metabolism and RNA and protein synthesis in the nerve cell bodies have also been determined in this way. Many molecular studies aimed at identifying genes and gene products involved in neural development use the powerful methods of recombinant DNA technology. Gene expression can also be analysed histologically using suitable RNA probes on tissue sections (*in situ* hybridisation). The effects of aberrant expression of neural developmental genes can be examined in whole animals by, for example, the creation of transgenic mice (injecting the male pronucleus after fertilisation with copies of the gene in question) or transgenic flies (using transposable elements to insert single copies of the gene into the early embryonic genome). The analysis of genetic mutations at the molecular level has also been very useful.

Experimental design

Armed with technical expertise, what kinds of experiment can the developmental neurobiologists do? There are three basic designs.

1. *Description of events in the normal animal.* The first stage in any study is to observe to the limit of the techniques available what happens in the normal developing animal. Such phenomenological observations give clues to underlying cellular and subcellular mechanisms.

2. *Description of events after experimental manipulations.* An hypothesis about mechanisms acting in the intact animal can be tested by altering conditions in an experimental animal and comparing the observed outcome with that predicted by the hypothesis. Pro-

cedures for altering conditions include either removing or translo-cating nerves or their targets, cutting or crushing axons and allowing them to regenerate, and changing the level of substances (e.g. hormones, transmitters, growth factors) thought to be important for an observed developmental phenomenon. Obser-vations on development in animals with single gene mutations affecting the nervous system also belong to this category of experimental design.

3. *Analysis of events in tissues in vitro.* The study of development in organ or tissue culture offers the possibility of testing hypotheses by altering conditions in ways that are not practical *in vivo.* Conditions in culture are sufficiently different from those in the animal to leave a doubt about the relevance of events or relative importance of effects seen in culture to those seen in the animal. Nevertheless, the culture approach has been particularly valuable for demonstrating the importance of chemical factors in guiding neuron growth and in keeping neurons alive. It has also been useful in determining some of the mechanisms of synaptogenesis and neuronal differentiation.

Most publications report the results of work on a single animal species, chosen from considerations of economy, availability and ease of experi-mentation for the particular developmental phenomenon being studied. Generally, the findings should not be assumed to apply more widely until they are confirmed in other species.

Part 2

Genesis of nerve cells

Chapter 3

Origin and differentiation of nerve cell types

Introduction

In any one region of the nervous system there are usually distinct sets of neurons that differ in morphology, patterns of connections, transmitter synthesis and transmitter sensitivities. Cells of a given set can also carry distinct surface labels to allow the ordered patterns of connections between one region and another to be established. Taken together, these distinguishing characteristics comprise the phenotype of a neuron. Altogether there are probably hundreds of distinct nerve cell phenotypes in an individual animal.

The various phenotypes each have to be generated from uncommitted, dividing precursor cells, and there are in principle two distinct mechanisms that can achieve this (fig. 3.1). In lineage (or intrinsic) specification, an asymmetric cell division distributes some sort of cytoplasmic determinant unequally between the daughter cells and thereby confers different fates on distinct daughter cells and their descendants. In inductive (or extrinsic) specification, different fates are conferred on identical daughter cells by position-dependent cell-cell interactions. To determine the nature of the specification mechanism for individual cells, their precursors first have to

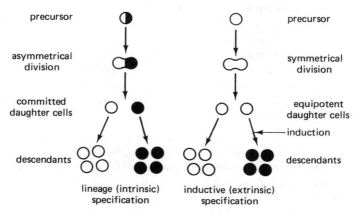

Fig. 3.1. Two mechanisms for specification of phenotype

15

be identified in the embryo, and then an appropriate experiment on the precursors has to be devised. The precursors are identified and their fates are traced by means of a cell marking or vital staining technique, or by direct observation if this is possible. Subsequent experiments include killing or removing some precursors, changing their position in the embryo, or changing their surrounding environment. If the fates of precursors are changed by these procedures, inductive specification is strongly indicated, and some clue to the nature of the inducing signal can be inferred by comparing the environments that induce different fates in the precursors. Unchanged fates mean either that specification is intrinsic or that fates have been determined prior to the experimental intervention. In some invertebrate systems, analysis of the effects of genetic mutations on cell lineage and fate has allowed the identification of some of the genes and gene products that direct these processes.

The neuronal phenotypes of invertebrates generally arise through lineages displaying invariant patterns of cell division. At first sight this might suggest the frequent operation of lineage-specification mechanisms, where fates are determined early and passed on by inheritance. Nevertheless, an increasing number of examples are being recognised in which these invariant patterns are actually the result of highly reproducible cell–cell interactions; in other words, both lineage and inductive specification mechanisms can contribute to the invariant lineages of invertebrates. For vertebrates, an inductive process operates at the time the first neuronal precursor cells arise from ectoderm and inductive cell–cell interactions appear to be responsible for specification of particular phenotypes at or after the final cell division. Similarly, the peripheral nervous system phenotypes derived from the neural crest appear to be induced by local environmental influences.

Specification in invertebrates

The small number of cells in invertebrates and their accessibility for observation and manipulation make it possible in some cases to identify specific individual neurons in the adult and in the embryo and to construct detailed lineages linking these cells. Certain organisms are also particularly amenable to the powerful methods of classical and molecular genetic analysis. In recent years, favoured systems have included the nematode worm, leech and fruitfly.

> *Nematode.* In the adult nematode worm, *Caenorhabditis elegans*, there are less than 1000 cells, and of these 302 are neurons. Direct observation of living cells using Nomarski optics in combination with analysis of serial electron micrographs has led to the identification of every cell in the animal in the post-hatching stages of development, and has revealed stereotyped, invariant patterns of cell division and differentiation (Sulston & Horvitz, 1977). For

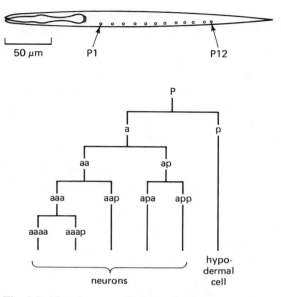

Fig. 3.2. Above: nematode immediately after hatching, showing position of the 12 P precursors of the ventral cord. Below: typical lineage of descendants of each P cell (a, anterior; p, posterior).

example, neurons of the ventral cord are generated by a stereotyped set of divisions of 12 precursors ('P' cells) aligned along the anterior–posterior axis of the animal (fig. 3.2). The daughter cells of a given P cell are all quite different in their phenotypes, but the daughter cells that arise by the same branch in each of the 12 lineages (lineally equivalent progeny) have similar phenotypes.

The invariant patterns of cell division and differentiation in the nematode arise not only from mechanisms operating through lineage ancestry; they are also due to highly reproducible cell–cell interactions. Investigation of the specification mechanism has been carried out by reconstructing lineages either in normal animals in which identified precursors have been killed with a laser microbeam, or in mutants with lineage abnormalities. Fates of surviving daughter cells are usually unchanged in these animals, even though they or their progeny occupy abnormal positions (Sulston & White, 1980). However, there are instances in the normal animal where individual precursor cells in identified small groups ('equivalence groups') choose among two or three similar but non-identical fates, the exact choice depending on interactions within the group or between the group and neighbouring cells. In the case of the 'P11/P12' equivalence group, for example, the normal P11 precursor adopts the P12 fate when the P12 precursor is ablated (Sulston & White, 1980) and gene products necessary for the expression of each of these fates have been identified (Sternberg, 1988). The *lin-12* locus has been shown to control cell fates in this and certain other nematode equivalence groups, as in the developing gonad. Interestingly, the *lin-12* product has some similarities to epidermal growth factor and its receptor, and to the product of the *Drosophila* neurogenic *Notch* locus (see below); it may be a transmembrane signalling protein mediating cell–cell interactions (Greenwald, 1989).

Leech. The longitudinal axis of the leech is established when five large ectodermal cells (teloblasts) on each side of the early embryo bud off long lines of cells (bandlets), which in turn give rise to the segmental ganglia of the nervous system. Cell lineage analysis has been undertaken using intracellular injection of HRP or fluorescent markers, showing that each ganglion derives cells from each of the five teloblast pairs through a stereotyped, invariant pattern of cell division. For a given ganglion, labelling of a single parent teloblast reproducibly stains a unique set of ganglion cells ('kinship group') of defined number, distribution and function (Stent & Weisblat, 1981). As for the nematode, a cell's lineage history is often a major determinant of its developmental fate, but there are also indications that local cell–cell interactions can be important. Eliminating the 'p' bandlet on one side by photoablation causes the neighbouring 'o' bandlet to adopt the p fate (Shankland, 1987). When born, the o and p blast cells appear to be developmentally equivalent; the divergence of their fates in the normal embryo is assumed to result from their different positions, perhaps exposing them to different environmental signals.

Fruitfly. Research at the molecular genetic level on the fruitfly, *Drosophila*, has been particularly successful in recent years in the attempt to define the links between early embryonic pattern formation and the determination of nerve cells. The fly nervous system consists of a brain and a chain of paired segmental ganglia, one pair for each body segment, and it is likely that the generation of the neural pattern is linked to the mechanisms that construct the segmented body plan. The embryonic ectoderm, from which the nervous system derives, is subdivided into segmental units by a hierarchical network of gene interactions. These interactions also determine the distinctive pattern of cell fates within each unit. Mutational analysis has led to the classification of the regulatory genes involved into *segmentation* genes, which construct the segmental pattern, and the *homeotic* genes, which confer individual identities upon each segment (see Akam, 1987, for review). Segmentation genes can be further subdivided into three groups:

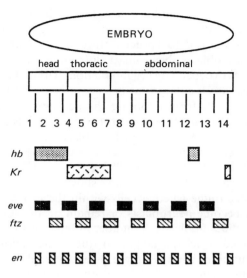

Fig. 3.3. Expression patterns of some of the segmentation genes during development of the *Drosophila* epidermis. The gap genes *hunchback (hb)* and *Kruppel (Kr)* are expressed in contiguous segmental domains, the segment polarity genes *fushitarazu (ftz)* and *even skipped (eve)* are expressed in alternating segmental domains and the segment polarity gene *engrailed (en)* is expressed in a part of each segmental domain.

gap genes, essential for the correct spatial expression of the *pair-rule* genes (transcribed in alternate segments); pair-rule genes in turn regulate the *segment-polarity* genes, which are required for pattern formation within each segment (fig. 3.3). The segmentation genes regulate the action of the homeotic genes. Many of these genes have now been cloned and sequenced, but the precise modes of operation of their products, which involve DNA-binding functions, remain to be clarified.

After gastrulation, the CNS develops from a layer of ventral ectoderm (the neurogenic region). About one-quarter (500) of these cells come to occupy the interior of the embryo, where a stereotyped pattern of further cell divisions takes place. Twenty five neuroblasts are generated for each half-segment; each neuroblast then acts as a stem cell, producing a chain of smaller cells called ganglion mother cells (GMCs), which divide once to produce two postmitotic neurons. Lineage analysis experiments in the grasshopper, whose nervous system has the same ground-plan as the fly, have shown that each neuroblast generates a characteristic, invariant set of GMCs and neurons (Doe & Goodman, 1985). A laser-ablated GMC cannot be replaced by a neighbouring cell, so GMCs are presumed to be determined by their ancestry from particular neuroblasts. Neuroblast differentiation, on the other hand, appears to depend on cell interactions within the neurogenic region. Once a cell enlarges to become a neuroblast, it inhibits neighbouring cells from adopting the neuroblast fate; instead, these cells either turn into non-neuronal support cells or die. But if the neuroblast is ablated it can be replaced by a neighbouring neurogenic cell (but not neuroblast), whose fate is that of the ablated cell (Doe & Goodman, 1985).

Transplantation experiments have shown that cell–cell interactions also determine whether cells within the neurogenic region move in to become neuroblasts or remain on the surface of the embryo as epidermoblasts. A number of 'neurogenic' genes have been identified which participate in these interactions; loss-of-function mutations in any of these genes cause all the neurogenic cells to adopt a neural fate and their normal operation is thought to generate an epidermalising signal to some of the neurogenic cells. Sequence analysis of two of these genes, *Notch* and *Delta*, shows that they encode transmembrane proteins whose extracellular domains comprise EGF-like repeats. As for *lin-12* (see above) this is suggestive of a signalling function, for example in a ligand–receptor interaction between neighbouring neurogenic cells that ultimately dictates their fates as nerve cell or epidermal cell respectively (fig. 3.4). Another gene complex, *achaete-scute* (AS-C), may be important in the further determination of the nerve cell pathway; deletion of the complex causes CNS degeneration, and AS-C transcription correlates closely with the stages of neuroblast segregation (Cabrera, Martinez Arias & Bate, 1987; Ghysen & Dambly-Chaudiere, 1989). How the products of the neurogenic genes interact with loci such as AS-C, and the role these loci play in generating the neuronal phenotype, are important questions for future research.

Some of the segmentation genes, such as the pair-rule genes *fushitarazu* (*ftz*) and *even-skipped* (*eve*), are expressed in the developing nervous system after the segmental pattern is established (fig. 3.5*a*), where they are likely to have a different role. If the neurogenic control element of *ftz* is removed, leaving its 'zebra' control element for segmentation intact, the later CNS expression can be abolished when the engineered gene is introduced into the fly germline (fig. 3.5*b*). In such embryos, the axon of one particular segmental motor neuron is found to take an abnormal course (Doe *et al.*, 1988). A similar abnormality is seen when *eve* expression is

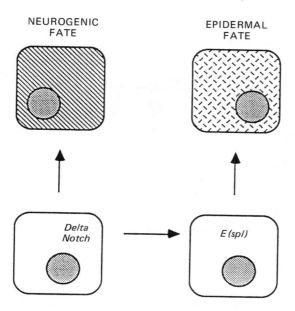

Fig. 3.4. The interaction between two neighbouring *Drosophila* neurogenic cells, which determines their fate as nerve cell and epidermal cell. The products of the neurogenic loci *Delta* and *Notch* (and several others), generated in the neuroblast, regulate *Enhancer of split* [E(spl)] expression in the epidermoblast. *E(spl)* products in turn regulate the genes necessary for epidermal development (after Campos-Ortega, 1988).

selectively abolished in this cell. The homeotic genes are also transcribed early during neurogenesis; as for the epidermis, they may determine segment-specific differentiation patterns. It is likely, therefore, that neuronal determination also involves the action of the segmentation and homeotic genes, which may interact with the neurogenic genes (Doe & Scott, 1988).

A final example of the utility of the fruitfly for understanding neural development comes from studies of photoreceptor differentiation in the compound eye (Tomlinson, 1988; Ready, 1989). The ommatidium, or unit eye, develops in a monolayer epithelium and comprises eight photoreceptor cells (R cells) and a complement of accessory cells. Using genetic markers to follow cell lineage, it has been shown that the fate of ommatidial cells does not depend on their lineage ancestry, even in their final divisions. In the mutant *sevenless*, one particular photoreceptor cell, R7, is absent; its precursor joins the developing ommatidial cluster on schedule, but becomes a non-neuronal cell instead. A genetically normal cell in

(a)

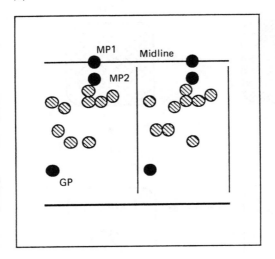

⊘ Cell which will give rise to *ftz*
producing cells.

● Cell which expresses *ftz*.

(b)

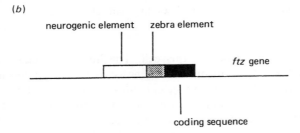

Fig. 3.5. (a) Expression of *ftz* in two adjacent segmental ganglia on one side of the *Drosophila* embryo. Cells which express *ftz*, or whose progeny will express *ftz*, are placed at defined positions and are surrounded by non-expressing cells. MP, midline precursor cell; GP, glial precursor cell. (b) Control of *ftz* gene expression is dependent on regulators which can bind to specific DNA 'elements' upstream of the gene. The zebra element is involved in controlling pair-rule segmental patterns during early development, and the neuroblast expression pattern in the CNS is determined by the neurogenic element.

the R7 position of an otherwise *sevenless* cluster will become R7, raising the possibility that the mutant R7 precursor cannot respond to some environmental signal that normally triggers it along the R7 differentiation pathway. Sequence analysis of the cloned *sevenless* gene predicts a transmembrane protein with a large external domain and an internal tyrosine kinase domain, which could act as a membrane receptor for the transduction of the signal to the nucleus. Another gene has been identified, *bride of sevenless* (*boss*), which is expressed in an adjacent cell, R8; when this gene is mutant, R7 again fails to appear. The *boss* gene may therefore code for the signal directing R7 development. Other genes critical to development in this system are now being identified. In summary, the favoured model for the specification of ommatidial cell fates invokes inductive interactions. Once a founder cell is designated, a chain reaction spreads to neighbouring, uncommitted cells; cell–cell interactions involving extracellular ligands and cell surface receptors activate the appropriate differentiation pathways in each cell.

Neural induction in vertebrates

For vertebrates, the importance of inductive processes in neural development has been recognised for many years, since the classical experiments of Spemann and Mangold (Spemann, 1938). By a process sometimes referred to as 'primary induction', the mesoderm lying beneath the dorsal ectoderm induces neural properties in it at the gastrulation stage of development (fig. 3.6). The mesoderm itself is thought to acquire its 'neuralising' capacity as it passes, during gastrulation, past the dorsal lip of the blastopore. The evidence for this scheme came from experiments in amphibian embryos. Transplantation of the blastopore region to another region of a host embryo could cause the development of a whole new nervous system from host ectoderm; mesoderm transplanted to the blastocoele of a host embryo could induce a second neural tube to form even if sited beneath ventral ectoderm (which does not normally give rise to nervous tissue); lastly, dorsal ectoderm transplanted to a host could give rise to a second neural tube only if the piece was taken after mesoderm had migrated in under it (i.e., after gastrulation) – otherwise it gave rise to epidermis.

The nature of the inducing signal passed from the mesoderm to ectoderm has remained elusive. After many years of research, including *in vitro* studies in which mixtures of ectoderm, mesoderm, cell extracts and a variety of chemicals have been tested, the consensus is that induction is likely to be mediated by diffusible agents from the mesoderm (Saxen, 1980), and that regional differentiation into forebrain, midbrain, hindbrain and spinal cord may depend upon the length of time the ectoderm is in contact with these agents. In amphibian embryos the mesoderm is itself induced,

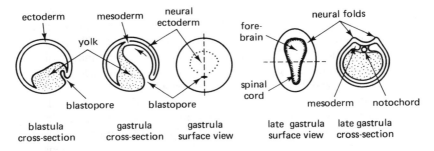

Fig. 3.6. Development of neural ectoderm (dashed lines show planes of section).

before neural induction, by cell interactions between the animal and vegetal cells of the blastula. In this case, inducing factors have been identified that are related to well-characterised peptide growth factors such as basic fibroblast growth factor and transforming growth factor beta (Smith, 1989). Whether neural induction is mediated by similar interactions is unknown; recent experiments in amphibian embryos suggest that the critical interaction may actually begin before movement of the mesoderm under the ectoderm (Dixon & Kintner, 1989), and that the dorsal ectoderm, as assayed by expression of a neural marker gene, is to some extent predetermined in its ability to respond appropriately to neural induction (Sharpe, Fritz & DeRobertis, 1987).

Specification of phenotypes in the vertebrate CNS

An important step towards understanding specification in the vertebrate CNS requires a description of the sequence of cell divisions leading to the final cell types for any particular CNS region. This has been undertaken recently for a variety of sites in the CNS with the use of retrovirus labelling or intracellular dye to identify clones descended from single cells and also with immunohistochemistry to examine the pattern of expression of antigens specific to neurons and glia during development. In the rat retina, individual virally-labelled clones (of five cells or less) were found to contain almost any combination of retinal nerve cell types – rods, bipolar cells, amacrine cells – as well as specialised glia (Turner & Cepko, 1987). This suggests that cell fates are determined extrinsically after the final mitosis, although an intrinsic mechanism cannot be completely ruled out. Clones of cells labelled with retrovirus at an early stage in the development of the chick optic tectum contained neurons, glia, and mixtures of these, indicating that some neuronal and glial phenotypes had diverged at the time their precursors were labelled (Sanes, 1989a). Divergence of neuronal and glial lines in the monkey forebrain was suggested by the observation that antibodies to a glial-specific protein bound to a subpopulation of the dividing cells in the ventricular (mitotic) zone (Levitt, Cooper & Rakic,

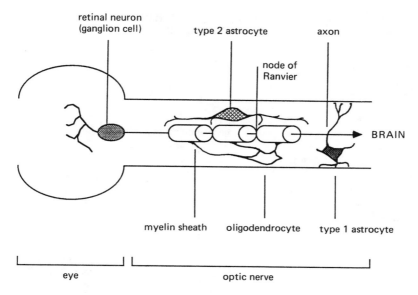

Fig. 3.7. Cell components of the rat optic nerve. Type 1 astrocytes provide a glial framework, oligodendrocytes myelinate the retinal ganglion cell axons, and type 2 astrocytes contact the axons at nodes of Ranvier (after Alberts *et al.*, 1989).

1981). Virally-labelled clones in the mouse cerebral cortex were almost exclusively neuronal or glial (Sanes, 1989*a*), and the type and distribution of the phenotypes in each clone was consistent with the manner in which cells are known to be generated in the cortex (see Chapter 4). In the chick hindbrain, precursor cells marked with fluorescent dye generally produced only one neuronal phenotype after a final few divisions, indicating a divergence of the neuronal phenotypes at the time of labelling (Keynes & Lumsden, 1990). The only generalisation that can be made from these disparate observations is that at some (but not all) sites in the CNS, the decision as to whether a cell is to be neural or glial is made well before the final mitosis. The mechanisms determining specific neuronal phenotypes are as yet unclear. It is worth noting that one glial population, the microglia, derives not from the neural epithelium but from the mesoderm, migrating into the CNS during early development; in keeping with their phagocytic function, microglia share a number of surface markers in common with peripheral macrophages (Perry & Gordon, 1988).

The mechanisms controlling cell fates in the CNS can also be studied *in vitro*, with the great advantage that the cell environment can be manipulated more precisely than *in vivo*. This approach has been taken successfully by Raff and colleagues, with an analysis of glial cell differentiation in the rat optic nerve (Raff, 1989). Three different glial types and their precursors can be distinguished on the basis of characteristic antibody staining patterns:

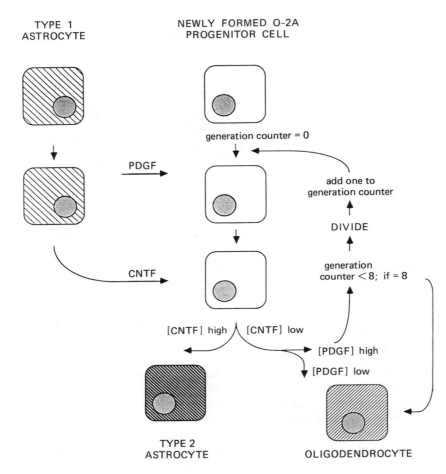

Fig. 3.8. Flow chart for glial differentiation in the rat optic nerve (after Alberts *et al.*, 1989).

oligodendrocytes (responsible for myelination), and type 1 and type 2 astrocytes (fig. 3.7). Oligodendrocytes and type 2 astrocytes develop postnatally from a bipotential precursor, the O-2A progenitor cell, while type 1 astrocytes develop before birth from a different precursor. *In vitro*, the presence of type 1 astrocytes drives the O-2A precursors through a specific number of cell cycles before their terminal differentiation; this process appears to be mediated by the release from the astrocytes of platelet-derived growth factor (PDGF). Whether the O-2A progenitor then becomes an oligodendrocyte or a type 2 astrocyte depends, in turn, on the presence of another growth factor produced by the type 1 astrocyte, ciliary neurotrophic factor (CNTF), which induces the type 2 differentiation pathway. In the absence of CNTF only oligodendrocytes are produced (fig. 3.8). Specific cell differentiation in this system is seen, therefore, to be the outcome of an intricate interaction between environmental signals and cell-autonomous behaviour.

A further aspect of neuronal phenotype that has been studied is the development of neuron-specific membrane properties. Cells of the vertebrate neural plate *in vivo* and *in vitro* develop action potentials dependent first on Ca^{2+} then on Na^+ and then become sensitive to neurotransmitter (Spitzer, 1981). It has also been shown that neuronal differentiation in amphibians is dependent on the proper functioning of the sodium pump at a critical developmental stage (Warner, 1985). Cells are coupled by low resistance junctions around the time specification of some neurons occurs, and it will be interesting to determine whether such coupling is necessary for phenotype specification.

Pattern formation in the vertebrate CNS
Are there any large-scale patterning mechanisms that could impart regional identity to different CNS areas? Or, put another way, how does a simple epithelial sheet generate the remarkable structural (and functional) diversity manifested by, for example, cerebral cortex and spinal cord? Subdivision by segmentation is commonly used in animal development to generate local anatomical variations in cell differentiation and pattern. Embryologists in the early part of this century were well aware of the existence of segmental swellings in the epithelium of the developing neural tube, but the significance of these 'neuromeres' was obscure. Recent studies of neuromeres in the developing hindbrain ('rhombomeres') have shown that here the segmental pattern is matched by an underlying segmental pattern of neuronal differentiation; for example, in the sequence of branchiomotor nerves V (trigeminal), VII (facial) and IX (glossopharyngeal), the motor nucleus of V is produced exclusively by rhombomeres 2 and 3 (r2,3), that of VII by r4,5 and that of IX by r6,7. Pairs of segments are matched to each adjacent branchial arch (Lumsden & Keynes, 1989) (fig. 3.9).

The development of the rhombomere pattern resembles the development of segmental patterns in the fruitfly. Like the boundaries of insect segments, the rhombomere boundaries are zones of lineage restriction that proliferating clones are unable to cross (Fraser *et al.*, 1990). Moreover, the expression patterns of some of the mouse 'homeobox genes', which share a DNA sequence in common with certain segmentation and homeotic genes of *Drosophila*, also correspond to the rhombomere pattern in early mouse embryos (fig 3.9; Wilkinson *et al.*, 1989). Together with the observation (see above) that lineage ancestry may play a role in determining cell fates in the hindbrain, these findings suggest that the mechanisms controlling the development of this region of the vertebrate CNS could be

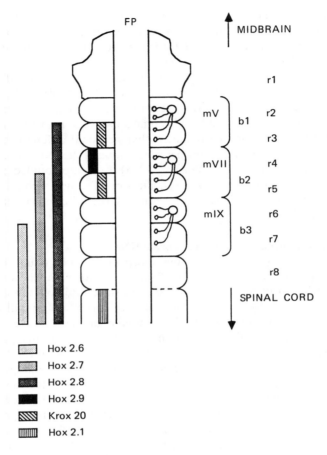

FP

MIDBRAIN

r1

mV
b1
r2

r3

mVII
b2
r4

r5

mIX
b3
r6

r7

r8

SPINAL CORD

Hox 2.6
Hox 2.7
Hox 2.8
Hox 2.9
Krox 20
Hox 2.1

Fig. 3.9. Arrangement of rhombomeres (r1–r8), branchial arches (b1–b3) and branchiomotor cranial nerves (mV, trigeminal; mVII, facial; mIX, glossopharyngeal) in the developing hindbrain of higher vertebrates. The exit points of mV, mVII and mIX lie in alternate segments r2, r4 and r6. On the left are shown the boundaries of expression of certain mouse homeobox genes (Hox 2.1, 2.6–2.9), and those of another gene whose product is predicted to bind DNA (Krox 20). These boundaries correspond to the rhombomere boundaries. FP, midline floorplate.

similar in principle to those controlling segmental development in the fly. Whether segmentation is important for the development of other CNS regions is unresolved. Neuromeres can also be seen in the fore- and midbrains, but their importance is not clear (Keynes & Lumsden, 1990). The spinal cord of higher vertebrates is not segmented; the repeat pattern of peripheral spinal nerves is caused by segmentation in the neighbouring mesoderm (Keynes & Stern, 1988).

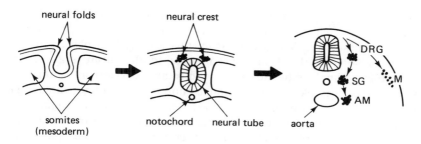

Fig. 3.10. Formation and migration of the neural crest at the level of somites 18–24, producing dorsal root ganglia (DRG), sympathetic ganglia (SG), adrenomedullary cells (AM) and melanocytes (M).

The derivatives of the neural crest

The neural crest forms as a transient structure when cells detach from the edge of the neural ectoderm at the time of closure of the neural tube. The cells migrate out into the periphery along well defined pathways (see later), and differentiate into neurons and glia of the peripheral nervous system (PNS), as well as craniofacial mesenchyme (contributing bone, cartilage and dentine) and melanocytes in the skin. Some cells of the cranial PNS also derive from epithelial thickenings (placodes) of the cephalic ectoderm (Le Douarin, 1986*b*).

Over the years, the neural crest has provided an outstanding example of the importance of environmental interactions in the determination of neuronal phenotype. A major contribution has come from Le Douarin and her colleagues, who have used the so-called xenoplastic grafting method for establishing lineages (Le Douarin, 1982, 1986*a*). In this technique tissues from quail embryos, the cells of which contain a prominent nucleolus, are transplanted to chick embryos. The resulting chimaeras develop normally and the graft and host cells or their descendants are readily distinguished by light or electron microscopy. Experiments in which small amounts of crest are transplanted to embryos of the same age and to the same level of the crest (isochronic and isotopic grafts) show that particular ganglia and nerve plexuses in the peripheral nervous system arise from particular levels of the crest. Moreover, each level of the crest gives rise to several phenotypes; for example, crest from rostrocaudal levels opposite somites 18–24 gives rise to adrenomedullary cells as well as sympathetic and sensory ganglia and melanocytes (fig. 3.10).

Are the various phenotypes specified before, during or after the migration of the crest cells? One way to investigate this is to see whether crest transplanted between different rostrocaudal levels (heterotopic grafting) behaves according to its level of origin or according to its new, grafted level. The answer is that crest cells usually behave exactly like the crest they replace. For example, crest migrating from the level of somites 1–7 does not contribute to any sympathetic ganglia but instead invades the gut, where it expresses a parasympathetic phenotype (detectable by the presence of acetylcholinesterase). When crest from this level is transplanted to the region of somites 18–24 the cells migrate to the future sites of the sympathetic ganglia and adrenal medulla and develop an adrenergic phenotype (detectable by catecholamine fluorescence), but not cholinergic phenotype (Le Douarin & Teillet, 1974). The role of the environment in determining crest cell fates can be interpreted in two ways. First, individual crest cells could be pluripotent at the onset of migration, their final fates being induced by specific signals encountered in their environment. Second, the migrating (or grafted) crest population could encompass a range of individual cells already committed to individual fates; specific environments would then lead to the selective proliferation or survival of cells with the appropriate phenotype in the appropriate position.

Recent studies have shown clearly that crest precursors can be pluripotent. Taking an *in vitro* approach, Baroffio, Dupin & Le Douarin (1988) generated large clones (up to 20 000 cells) from single cranial crest cells by culturing them on layers of suitable feeder cells. Using a variety of antibody and histochemical markers they found that each clone could be highly heterogeneous, with both neuronal and non-neuronal phenotypes. A direct demonstration of pluripotentiality *in vivo* has been provided by lineage analysis of the avian trunk crest, using iontophoresis of a fluorescent marker dye to fill single parent cells just prior to their migration from the neural tube (Bronner-Fraser & Fraser, 1988). Clones derived from such cells could contain as many as four different cell types: sensory neurons, adrenomedullary cells, Schwann cells and pigment cells. There is evidence, nevertheless, that the premigratory crest does not comprise a uniform population of pluripotent cells. For example, cranial crest contributes to craniofacial mesenchymal tissues while trunk crest does not, but cranial crest grafted to the trunk level still gives rise to mesenchyme, suggesting that the mesenchymal phenotype is prespecified in cranial crest (Le Douarin, 1982). Again, nearly one quarter of fluorescently labelled clones in the experiments of Bronner-Fraser & Fraser (1988) were confined to the dorsal root ganglia.

Precisely when and how the various neuronal subpopulations (such as sympathoadrenal, parasympathetic and sensory) diverge from one another is under active investigation (see Anderson, 1989, for review). *In vitro* studies have allowed some of the relevant environmental signals to be characterised in certain cases, and a good illustration of this approach is provided by the experiments of Patterson and colleagues (Patterson, Potter & Furshpan, 1978). The transmitter phenotype of cultured sympathetic neurons can be switched from noradrenergic to cholinergic by medium conditioned by heart cells (Patterson & Chun, 1977), and this 'cholinergic factor' has turned out to be a cytokine known as leukaemia inhibitory factor (LIF) (Yamamori *et al.*, 1989). An attractive possibility is that the normal targets of sympathetic cholinergic innervation, such as sweat glands, induce cholinergic properties in the neurons by the release of this substance (Schotzinger & Landis, 1988). As a further example, chromaffin cell differentiation is dependent *in vitro* on the presence of glucocorticoid hormones, mimicking the presumed influence of the adrenal cortex *in vivo* (Doupe, Patterson & Landis, 1985).

Chapter 4

Neuron proliferation and migration in vertebrates

The invariant lineage programmes that generate the invertebrate CNS involve little active cell migration. Vertebrates, by contrast, have adopted a very different strategy to produce the large numbers of nerve cells required at specific locations in the CNS: most nerve cells are born close to the inner surface of the neural tube and have to migrate subsequently past other cells, born themselves at an earlier stage, to their final positions. As we have seen, the development of the vertebrate peripheral nervous system also involves the extensive migration of cells.

Zones of proliferation in the developing CNS and the movement of neurons from these zones to their final positions, were first described using the light microscope. The early neural tube appears as a columnar epithelium in which the cells extend from the inner (ventricular) to the outer (pial) surface. Mitoses occur at the ventricular surface, and between mitoses the nuclei migrate towards the pial surface (fig. 4.1). The first cells to become postmitotic migrate outwards and take up positions at well-defined levels. As the tube thickens the mitotic cells remain localised to its inner side, thereby defining the ventricular germinal zone.

The details of the subsequent phase of proliferation and migration have been determined with the aid of tritiated thymidine (^{3}H-T) autoradiography. Animals are exposed to ^{3}H-T at progressively later stages of development, and CNS sections are processed for autoradiography after a defined period of further development. Neurons completing their last round of DNA synthesis at the time of exposure to ^{3}H-T are heavily labelled in all

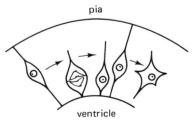

Fig. 4.1. Migration of nuclei between mitosis and after the last mitosis in early neural tube.

subsequent autoradiographs, while postmitotic neurons remain free of label. The time and place of 'birth' of each type of neuron and its subsequent movement can thus be reconstructed.

Phylogenetically older neurons, for example Rohon-Beard cells, are amongst the first to be born (Lamborghini, 1980). The largest neurons in any given region of the mature nervous system (e.g. pyramidal cells of cerebral cortex) are also amongst the first to become postmitotic, apparently because the largest neurons, which have the longest axons, have to reach their distant targets when the embryo is still small. The smaller local circuit neurons are generated next, followed finally by the glia, many of which are able to divide even in the mature nervous system (Lewis, 1968; Ludwin, 1984).

In the regions of the brain that have a laminar structure (such as the cerebral and cerebellar cortices), postmitotic cells migrate continually to the more superficial levels, so that the cell layers are laid down 'inside-out' (Angevine & Sidman, 1961); in nuclear regions (e.g. thalamus, hypothalamus), on the other hand, cells accumulate in an 'outside-in' sequence (fig. 4.2) (Rakic, 1977a). In the mammalian forebrain a second proliferative zone, the subventricular germinal zone, develops above the ventricular germinal zone. Electron microscopic reconstructions in monkeys suggest that the radial migration of postmitotic neurons from these zones is guided by radially-oriented glial cells, which extend from the ventricular to the pial surface (Rakic, 1972). This has led Rakic (1988) to propose the 'radial unit hypothesis'. It is suggested that discrete ventricular proliferative units exist, whose progeny, numbering in the Rhesus monkey between 80 and 120 neurons, migrate along a single or a small group of radial glial cells. These units provide a 'proto-map' of future cortical areas, and could be the basis of the well-known columnar organisation of the adult cortex.

The aspect of phenotype that determines how far a neuron migrates in the developing cortex appears to be determined within the ventricular zone before migration. When ³H-T-labelled ventricular cells from ferret embryos, destined for cortical layers 5 and 6, are grafted into the telencephalon of older (neonatal) hosts, many still differentiate and project as layer

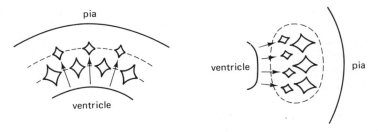

Fig. 4.2. 'Inside-out' assembly of laminar structures (left) and 'outside-in' assembly of nuclei (right).

5/6 neurons, and not as the layer 2/3 neurons being generated in the host brain (McConnell, 1989). Again, in a mutant mouse, 'reeler', in which the cortical layers are malpositioned, neurons differentiate according to their origins rather than their new, abnormal locations (Caviness, 1982).

In the cerebellum and the dentate gyrus of the hippocampus a proliferative layer develops at the pial surface, when dividing cells migrate here from nearby proliferative regions. In the dentate gyrus, postmitotic cells from this layer penetrate radially to deeper layers, coming to rest in an outside (oldest)-in (youngest) sequence (Schlessinger, Cowan & Gottlieb, 1975). In the cerebellum, the granule cells that arise from the external germinal layer are guided to deeper layers by glia (Bergmann glial cells), and the remaining neurons are generated in an inside-out sequence (Rakic, 1971; Altman, 1972). Progress has been made recently in characterising adhesion molecules that may mediate the migration of cerebellar granule cells on the Bergmann glia, using *in vitro* assays (Hatten & Mason, 1986). Migration is inhibited by antibodies against two such components, 'adhesion molecule on glia' (Antonicek, Persohn & Schachner, 1987) and 'astrotactin' (Edmondson *et al.*, 1988). Other adhesion molecules such as cytotactin/tenascin may also play a role (Chuong, Crossin & Edelman, 1987) (see Chapter 6 for further discussion of adhesion molecules).

Regional differences in cell division rate probably contribute to the complex folding of the neural tube as development proceeds, and to the later formation of cortical gyri and sulci (Richman *et al.*, 1975). The factors determining such differences, as well as local variations in cell number, are not well understood. To achieve the correct ratio of glial cells to axons during development it may be that neurons control glial mitosis. At least two glial mitogens have been characterised: one is surface-bound on sensory and sympathetic neurons (Ratner *et al.*, 1988), the second is a protein (glial growth factor) extractable from brain and pituitary, which triggers Schwann cell and fibroblast proliferation *in vitro* (Brockes & Lemke, 1981; Brockes, 1984). It is also possible that neurotransmitters have mitogenic roles during development (Hanley, 1989; Ashkenazi, Ramachandran & Capon, 1989).

The migration of neural crest cells along specific pathways in the periphery is probably controlled by adhesive interactions between the crest cell surface and local extracellular matrix molecules. Fibronectin provides an adhesive substrate for crest migration *in vitro*, and its effects can be modulated by cytotactin/tenascin (Halfter, Chiquet Ehrismann & Tucker, 1989); cranial crest migration *in vivo* is inhibited by the injection of antibodies to a number of adhesion molecules, including a laminin–heparan sulphate proteoglycan complex and integrins (Bronner-Fraser, 1986, 1987, 1988). Trunk crest cells migrate preferentially into the cranial half of each somite to form the segmental dorsal root ganglia and sympathetic ganglia; this preference is likely to result from a combination of adhesive interactions in the cranial half-somite and inhibitory interactions with cells of the caudal half-somite (Keynes & Stern, 1988; Stern *et al.*, 1989). For migrating cells in both CNS and PNS, it is still unclear exactly how such interactions are translated into the membrane and cytoskeletal changes that actually move the cell; nor is it clear what determines the cessation of movement at appropriate positions.

Conclusion to Part 2

Our understanding of the early stages of brain development, which only a decade ago was fragmentary, has improved considerably. Rapid progress has been made in the comparatively simple nervous systems of invertebrates. Here, specification is dependent on both lineage ancestry and on cell–cell interactions, probably to differing degrees in different systems. The techniques of molecular genetics are allowing a detailed analysis of the underlying mechanisms. In vertebrates, the importance of environmental signals in determining cell fates had long been suspected and has been confirmed using newly developed techniques for following cell lineage. Studies *in vitro* have identified some of these signals at the molecular level, and have enabled factors involved in the migration of neurons and neural crest cells to be characterised.

Part 3

Establishing connections

Part-I

Simplifying Connections?

Chapter 5

Axon and dendrite growth

Axon growth cones

Cajal recognised that axon growth occurred at the terminal enlargement of the axon that could be seen in silver stained preparations of embryonic tissue and he coined the term 'cone of growth' for this structure (see Cajal, 1928, p.363). Growth cones were observed subsequently by Harrison (1910) in the first tissue cultures to be established successfully and later by Speidel (1942) in living tadpole tails. More recent observations have been carried out on the growth cones of sensory or autonomic neurons from chick or rat embryonic ganglia in tissue culture. Direct observation of growth cones in intact animals is also possible (Harris, Holt & Bonhoeffer, 1987). Biochemical studies have been carried out on growth cones isolated from foetal brains (Pfenninger, 1986).

Electron microscopy has shown that the growth cone contains mitochondria, vesicles, microfilaments and microtubules (fig. 5.1). Extending beyond it are fine outgrowths called filopodia (or microspikes), which are extended and withdrawn rapidly for distances of up to 50μm. The filopodia contain microfilaments which can be stained with antibodies raised against actin and myosin (Letourneau, 1981).

Attachment of growth cones to substrates is a vital part of axonal growth and occurs mainly at points of adhesion beneath the filopodia (Letourneau, 1979). There have been several clear demonstrations that growth cones grow better on surfaces to which they can adhere strongly and that they show a graded preference for these surfaces in culture; they prefer, for example, polylysine to collagen, and collagen to agar (Letourneau, 1975). A particularly favourable substrate found in the extracellular matrix is laminin (Carbonetto, Evans & Cochard, 1987; Montell & Goodman, 1988) and neurons, like other cells, possess receptors called integrins that recognise it (Ignatius & Reichardt, 1988). Laminin and other material released from cells is an excellent growth substrate for axons when it becomes bound to the surface of a culture dish (e.g. Adler *et al.*, 1981), and this may explain why axons growing out from explants of different ganglia in culture turn selectively towards explants of their own target tissues (e.g. Ebendal & Jacobson, 1977). Axons also tend to adhere to the surfaces of

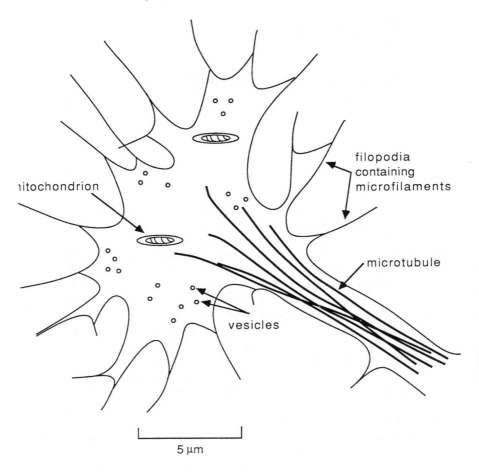

Fig. 5.1. Diagram of a growth cone.

glial cells or other axons as they grow *in vivo* and *in vitro*. In the case of growth on astrocytes several adhesion molecules, such as N-cadherin and N-CAM, may be involved (see section in Chapter 6) in addition to molecules recognised by integrin (Neugebauer *et al.*, 1988). Antibodies to N-CAM disrupt the ordered growth of retinal axons within the optic nerve of the chick (Thanos, Bonhoeffer & Rutishauer, 1984) demonstrating that bundling together of axons as they grow (fasciculation) helps to develop the normal tidy appearance of neural pathways in the adult and is achieved by surface molecules carried on growth cones. Selective guidance of particular groups of axons could be achieved theoretically by quite weak preferential affinities (Whitelaw & Cowan, 1981; Bennett & Robinson, 1989) and there is *in vitro* evidence that this is true (Walter *et al.*, 1987).

Growth cones will also turn towards higher concentrations of some diffusible substances (chemotropism), in particular Nerve Growth Factor (NGF), and there is evidence that this response is mediated by a rise in the filopodial Ca^{2+} concentration (Gundersen & Barrett, 1980) which might increase rates of filament or membrane assembly. Factors other than NGF emanating only from the appropriate target tissue have also been shown to attract sensory axons of the mouse maxillary nerve *in vitro* (Lumsden & Davies, 1983).

These observations suggest that axon guidance *in vivo* could be determined by chemically labelled substrates or by gradients of diffusible substances. Growth cones can be steered *in vitro* by weak electric fields. Such fields could exist in the embryo and may contribute to axon guidance but in a non-specific way (Jaffe & Poo, 1979). The variable rate at which growth cones advance might be associated with their capacity to secrete proteases (Monard, 1988) and so fashion for themselves an appropriate environment. An additional source of information to axons seeking their targets may come from material which prevents rather than encourages growth (Patterson, 1988). A striking example of this is the way in which motor axons leaving the spinal cord are channelled into the cranial half of the somite by an inhibitory factor present in the caudal half (Davies *et al.*, 1990). Direct inhibition of axon regrowth may also obtain following injury in the adult mammalian CNS when regenerating axons may be halted by products of mature oligodendrocytes (Schwab & Caroni, 1988).

The morphology of the growth cone varies as it grows towards its target. In particular, when growth slows the complexity of the cone increases (Bastiani *et al.*, 1985; Tosney & Landmesser, 1985). This occurs at points in the developing pathway where the growth cone has to 'decide' which direction to take. Whether the change in morphology is a cause or effect of slower growth, and what signals the change, are as yet unknown. The local mechanisms that determine if a growth cone divides to produce new branches are also unknown, but might depend on the pattern of adhesive molecules.

Mechanism of axonal elongation

The means by which additional membrane is added to the growth cone to enable it to advance is not certain, but a model has been proposed in which membrane vesicles, carried first into the growth cone by rapid axonal transport from the cell body, are then transported to the tips of the filopodia by an interaction between a myosin-like protein on the vesicle surface and the actin in the microfilaments (Bray, 1973). It seems that filopodial protrusion occurs at random from the growth cone, possibly powered by the rapid polymerisation of actin into rods. These actin filaments may then be pulled back into the body of the growth cone by an interaction with myosin located beneath the membrane. This will lead to retraction unless the actin can be anchored indirectly to the substrate. This could happen by means of a receptor in the membrane (e.g. integrin)

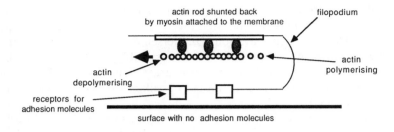

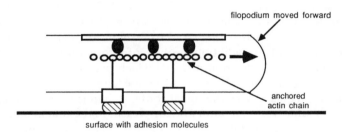

Fig. 5.2. Possible modes of retraction (above) or advance (below) of growth cone filopodium on an adhesive surface.

attaching to a molecule bound to the extracellular matrix and at the same time to the actin by means of a linking molecule (Mitchison & Kirschner, 1988; fig. 5.2). Then the surface membrane would be advanced.

Until recently it was thought that material for extension of microtubules was added to existing microtubules at the cell body, the whole array of microtubules being 'pushed' forward, as it were, from behind (Lasek, 1982). However, there is now evidence both for microtubules (Bamburg, Bray & Chapman, 1986) and neurofilaments (Nixon, 1987) that assembly occurs at the distal growing end from transported subunits travelling at the rate of slow transport along an essentially stationary framework of microtubules (Mitchison & Kirschner, 1988). The rate of growth cone advance can be faster than the rate at which neurofilaments can extend, so that these get progressively left behind (Tetzlaff & Bisby, 1989).

While their axons and dendrites are extending, neurons make large amounts of special growth-associated proteins (GAPs) that are not made at all or only in very small amounts at other times (Skene, 1984). Amongst these are GAP-43 (synonyms include B50, F1, pp46 and p57) which is a substrate for protein kinase-C and is concentrated in the axonal but not dendritic growth cone (Goslin *et al.*, 1988). The amounts of tubulin and actin being made also increase. The gene for class II β-tubulin is expressed at a particularly high level during growth (Hoffman, 1988), as is the gene for the Tα1 subunit of tubulin (Miller *et al.*, 1989) and the gene for actin (Tetzlaff, Bisby & Kreutzberg, 1988).

Intercalated growth

Axons reach their targets long before an animal has reached full size. It follows that as the animal grows extra material must be incorporated into axons so that they can keep contact with their synapses. Rather little is known about this, but the stimulus seems likely to be tension (Campenot, 1985). Axons also grow in diameter and new membrane must again be added. As the diameter increases the number of neurofilaments increases but the number of microtubules does not change (Hoffman, 1988).

Neuronal polarity

Foetal hippocampal neurons explanted before the development of any cell processes subsequently develop in culture an approximately normal morphology (Banker & Cowan, 1979). Careful examination shows that all processes grow initially at the same rate but eventually one accelerates and becomes the axon (Goslin & Banker, 1989). This cell process gradually acquires the biochemical properties unique to axons and the other branches acquire those unique to dendrites. One particularly interesting difference is the organisation of microtubules: in axons, these are polarised with the so-called plus end, where new subunits are most easily added, at the growing tip, but in dendrites there are microtubules of both polarities. This difference may help to account for the different organelles found in dendrites and axons (Black & Baas, 1989). It seems that ribosomes and Golgi bodies travel along microtubules preferentially from their plus to their minus ends (fig. 5.3). As only dendrites have microtubules of such polarity, this could explain why they, and not axons, have such organelles.

If the budding axon is pruned shorter than the other branches, one of these, usually the longest, takes over as the axon (Goslin & Banker, 1989). Thus the neuronal polarity first acquired is not immutable and this suggests that, *in vivo*, interactions with the surroundings could help to generate the stereotyped polarity of neurons. A parallel is seen in epithelial sheets, where the cells become polarised by interactions with other cells (Rodriguez-Boulan & Nelson, 1989). One of the first signs of developing neuronal polarity is the concentration of GAP-43 exclusively in the axon and its disappearance from the dendrites (Sargent, 1989 and Goslin *et al.*, 1988).

Dendrite growth

Structures analogous to axonal growth cones can be identified at the tips of developing dendrites in the light and electron microscopes (e.g. Morest, 1969; Skoff & Hamburger, 1974). Guidance of these dendritic growth cones appears to be influenced by the surrounding tissues. For example the dendrites of Purkinje cells in the cerebellum do not develop their normal

dendrites

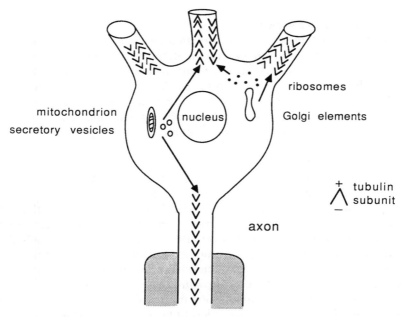

Fig. 5.3. Development of neuronal 'polarity'. Microtubules in axons have only one polarity and so do not transport ribosomes and Golgi elements.

fan-like shape and are stunted in mice lacking parallel fibres (Rakic, 1975). Thus the parallel fibres appear to stimulate and direct the growth of the dendrites of these cells. The mechanism underlying the control of this growth is not known, but it probably involves contact between the parallel fibres and the filopodia of the dendritic growth cones.

Functional synaptic input in addition to simple synaptic contact may play an important part in dendrite growth. The effects of complete block of activity on dendrite growth are not known, but a reduction in activity in the visual cortex of dark-reared animals leads to a failure in development of dendritic spines on pyramidal neurons (Valverde, 1967). Another clear example of the importance of afferent input in controlling dendritic development is seen in the Mauthner cell of the fish (Kimmel, 1982) where removal of the vestibular input stunts the lateral dendrite's growth. Even in adult animals elimination of input can cause dendritic changes (Jones & Thomas, 1962), from which it may be concluded that the 'skeletal' framework of the neuron (the neurofilaments and microtubules) is normally maintained in a state of equilibrium rather than being fixed permanently. Repeated observation of living neurons in autonomic ganglia of mice reveals that the dendritic tree is normally undergoing continuous remodelling (Purves & Hádley, 1985). A striking example of remodelling has been described in a larval motoneuron of the tobacco hornworm moth when the larval nervous system undergoes transformation to the adult form (Truman & Reiss, 1976).

Hormones can also influence the growth of dendrites of appropriate neurons: in a nucleus controlling song in the male canary (the singing sex) the neurons have cell bodies and dendrites that are twice the size of those in the female, but androgens can cause large neurons to develop in the female (Konishi & Gurney, 1982).

For some neurons certain aspects of dendritic growth are not dependent on environmental factors but are determined by factors intrinsic to the neuron. Thus the direction of growth of dendrites of the pyramidal neurons in the cerebral cortex appears, surprisingly, to be set by the direction of the axis of the cell body rather than by any external influences (Globus & Scheibel, 1967). Immature hippocampal neurons when dispersed in culture will develop reasonably normal primary dendritic branches (Banker & Cowan, 1979). The development of tertiary branches (spines), complete with postsynaptic densities, can occur on Purkinje cells in the absence of the presynaptic parallel fibres (Rakic, 1975). An interesting opportunity to study the minutiae of factors controlling neuronal shape was taken by Macagno, Lopresti & Levinthal (1973) and Goodman (1978) in partheno-genetically produced crustacea and insects. In these isogenic individuals the intrinsic factors controlling nerve cell shape and the extrinsic environment should be identical. Identifiable nerve cells in different individuals were found to be very similar in nearly every respect and differed only in the finest terminal branch pattern, whose shape depends presumably on chance events.

Numbers of dendrites in a particular population of neurons vary from species to species. Purves and his colleagues have pointed out that the range of animal sizes far exceeds the range of numbers of neurons, i.e. where there is a fiftyfold difference in size there may only be a three or fourfold difference in neuronal number. Larger animals seem to compensate for relatively low neuronal numbers by having neurons with bigger dendritic trees and axons with more terminal branches (Purves *et al.*, 1986, 1988; Purves, 1988). Voyvodic (1989*a*) has shown that sympathetic neurons in the superior cervical sympathetic ganglion of the rat develop very large dendritic trees if there is more target tissue for them to innervate and conversely that their dendritic arbours shrink if there is less target tissue. Feedback signals from the target (which in the case of the sympathetic neurons is likely to be Nerve Growth Factor – see Chapter 8) are the most important controller of the size of dendritic trees.

It is clear, then, that the overall growth of dendrites and the final shape of a given neuron is determined by a combination of intrinsic and extrinsic factors.

Chapter 6

Axon guidance and target recognition

Introduction

The gross patterns of peripheral nerves and nerve tracts in the CNS are usually identical in different animals of the same species and very similar in animals of related species, so it is obvious that some form of guidance must operate when axons first grow out through their surrounding tissues. When growth cones arrive in their target area they are always confronted with several different cell types, so it is also obvious that some form of target recognition must exist to permit synapses to form in the long term only between appropriately matched types of cells. Closer examination of the axonal connections normally reveals additional precise point-to-point mappings connecting cells from a particular region in the source nucleus with cells in a particular part of the target nucleus or region. This further refinement could be established if the outgrowing axons were collected in an orderly manner at their starting point and travelled together without change of relative position to their target area; alternatively, labels specific to their place of origin could be carried by axons and be used in specific guidance or recognition mechanisms.

Experiments in which regrowing axons in adults or embryonic outgrowing axons are challenged with different tissues or targets have revealed that the common sense predictions outlined above are borne out in practice. Evidence exists in nearly all the systems that have been examined for a variety of cues to assist in the construction of correct and orderly connections. These include appropriately placed non-specific guidance channels, active sorting of axons as they travel by means of specific cell-attached or substrate-bound signals, chemotropic signals and specific target recognition mechanisms that allow cell-specific and place-specific connections to form. The relative importance of each of these potential mechanisms varies from system to system. In some of them it seems that correct connections can form even if one of the normal cues is removed; in others all cues must be present. In this chapter the evidence for the existence of a range of different guidance cues and for the existence of specific target labelling is followed by examples of specific systems.

It should be emphasised that the guidance and target recognition systems do not set up the final wiring pattern of the nervous system; fine tuning of the initial connections occurs at a later stage, with the first crop of nerve terminals competing for long-term occupation of sites. The outcome depends upon a variety of factors but one is the degree of matching of chemospecific labels that set up the first, more crude, projection (see Chapter 9).

Non-specific guidance pathways

Transplantation experiments designed to make axons grow through tissues they would not normally encounter have provided convincing evidence for non-specific guidance pathways in the central and peripheral nervous systems. In general, the 'foreign' axons grow reproducibly along pathways that would be the sites of the normal nerve tracts in the tissue. For example, axons from transplanted retina will follow certain tracts in the spinal cord (Katz & Lasek, 1978), and axons from inappropriate spinal nerves will grow into transplanted limbs and produce the same gross pattern of peripheral nerves as in a normal limb (e.g. Summerbell & Stirling, 1981). It seems likely that many of the major tracts in the nervous system are non-specific and it has been suggested that the pathways are determined in a regular geometric pattern on the neural plate (Katz, Lasek & Nauta, 1980).

Non-specific guidance could be provided by blood vessels or by boundaries between different types of tissue. Specialised structures that develop apparently for the sole purpose of axon guidance can also occur: a 'sling' of glial cells between the cerebral hemispheres plays an essential role in the formation of the corpus callosum, because the corpus callosum does not develop in mice in which the sling has been sectioned, and the sling does not develop in marsupials or mutant mice lacking a corpus callosum in the adult (Silver *et al.*, 1982). In some instances guidance can be attributed to areas of low cell density in the tissue. For example, in the spinal cord cell-free channels can be demonstrated between the glial cells along the sites of future tracts (Singer, Norlander & Egar, 1979).

Specific guidance mechanisms

Active guidance cues can be inferred to exist if a bundle of axons makes abrupt changes in its direction of growth at particular and reproducible points along its pathway, especially if axons with different origins make different choices of direction. Such choice points can be further localised and studied by observing the effects of rotating or removing the region of the pathway in which they lie. This has been done by Landmesser and her colleagues who have studied the pathway from the spinal cord into the developing limb that is followed by the axons of motor neurons (Landmesser, 1984). They have found a region at the base of the limb (corresponding to the site of the adult nerve plexus) where motor axons, hitherto present in a more or less random order, are re-sorted into specific groups,

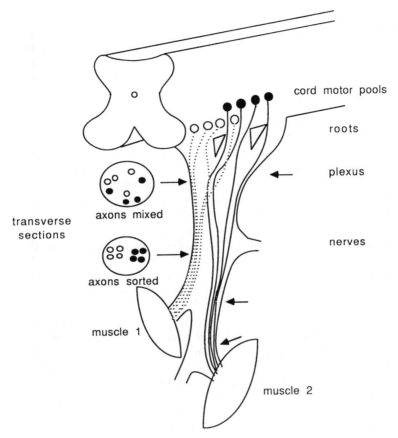

Fig. 6.1. Routes taken by motor axons into the limbs. Axons make 'decisions' about direction of growth in the plexus and where they leave the main nerve to enter their own muscle (arrows) (after Landmesser, 1984).

each group being destined for a particular muscle (fig. 6.1). Growth cones at this point on the pathway look different from those elsewhere (Tosney & Landmesser, 1985): they are larger and flatter and send out filopodia in many directions. It is at such places that bends develop in what would otherwise be a straight axonal trajectory. Electron microscopy of axonal contacts in these regions shows that mesenchymal cells in the region of the axon tips are dying but the axons themselves are not responsible for this (Tosney, Schroeter & Pokrzywinski, 1988). It appears that the axons are following a pattern of markers laid down in the mesenchyme that is linked in some way with necrosis of cells in discrete and reproducible sites. How this pattern is laid down is not known, and to explain the generation of enough markers to provide specific guides for the assembly of axons into nerves for each of the many muscles in the limb is a major puzzle. Whatever the cues may consist of they appear to work across species, for in chimeric preparations in which chick limb buds are transplanted to quails, the quail motor neurons innervate homologous muscles (Tanaka & Landmesser, 1986a).

In the vertebrate CNS too, active guidance regions are seen. A good example is provided by the optic pathway. In *Xenopus* embryos rotation of portions of the neuroepithelium in a clockwise or counter-clockwise direction makes the axons of retinal ganglion cells (fluorescently labelled so that the progress of individual axons can be followed *in vivo*) change the angle of their advance as they reach the rotated section of the pathway and then redirect towards their target again as they leave the rotated section (Harris, 1989). Furthermore, the well ordered axons of retinal ganglion cells re-sort themselves into a new order in the optic tract as they approach the tectum (e.g. Scholes, 1979). At this point in the pathway the glial environment of the cells changes but how this relates to the re-ordering is not clear (Maggs & Scholes, 1986). Further evidence that glial cells may contain important clues comes from an examination of the organisation of radial glial cells in the chick optic tectum and the relationship of the ingrowing optic axons to them. The optic axons grow across the tectum in a superficial layer and then plunge at right angles to this, travelling down beside the perpendicularly orientated radial glia towards the stratum griseum in which they find their synaptic partners (Vanselow *et al.*, 1989). The point at which different optic axons choose to make this change in direction is not randomly placed for they seem to peel off and descend in a highly ordered way.

Perhaps the best examples of active contact guidance are to be found in the developing insect CNS and PNS. Sensory axons growing into the CNS make sharp changes in direction at sites of particular cells, called 'stepping stones' by Bate (1976). Such sharp reproducible bends are not easily explained by chemotactic gradients or chemotropic attractants. Similar observations in the CNS of the grasshopper by Goodman and his colleagues point to discrete labels existing on pathways (Bastiani *et al.*, 1985). Individual axons arising from different neurons may initially run beside one another but at particular places they part company (fig. 6.2). The parting of the ways depends on the various axons possessing different surface labels that allow only certain axons to adhere to the existing scaffold of longitudinally running nerves, indeed only closely to one particular axon (Raper, Bastiani & Goodman, 1983). It seems that a given neuron can change the particular molecules it expresses as it develops (Harrelson & Goodman, 1988; Dodd & Jessell, 1988) so that as its axon elongates into a new environment it can make further specific choices about where to grow. Monoclonal antibodies raised against grasshopper neuroepithelium recognise unique subsets of developing grasshopper neurons (Goodman &

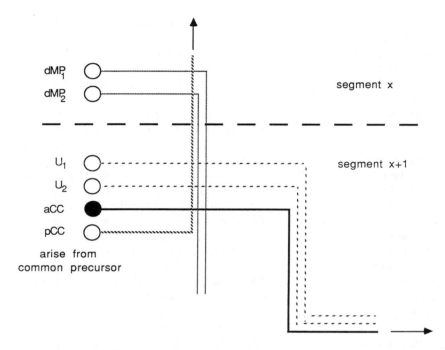

Fig. 6.2. Selective growth of axons in the insect. Axons from cells aCC and pCC make quite different 'decisions' about which direction to grow; aCC fasciculates with axons of U1 and U2, but pCC runs with axons of dMP1 and dMP2 (after Goodman & Bastiani, 1984).

Bastiani, 1984; Harrelson & Goodman, 1988). It is therefore likely that individual neurons and their axons and growth cones possess sets of surface molecules that are used to guide their own growth and that of other neurons in a very precise and unique way.

One of the mechanisms suggested for specific guidance is **chemotropism**: guidance by concentration gradients that exert an attractive influence on growth cones of a prospective synaptic partner. A striking, but artificial, demonstration of such chemotropism was provided by the effects of injections of Nerve Growth Factor (see Chapter 8) in large quantities into neonatal rat brains: the NGF apparently diffused down tissue spaces in the brain and spinal cord and caused a massive ingrowth of fibres from the sympathetic ganglia into the cord and up to the site of injection (Menesini-Chen, Chen & Levi-Montalcini, 1978). NGF itself is not, however, a good candidate as a specific chemotropic molecule for although it is a vital trophic substance for a wide range of neurons (Chapter 8), it is often not manufactured by target neurons until after they have become innervated (Davies, 1987). Furthermore, the innervating axons themselves do not become dependent on it until then. However, there is evidence that other, more specific, substances are manufactured and released at times that are appropriate to attract nearby axons. Lumsden & Davies (1983) have shown in *in vitro* experiments that epithelial cells of the second maxillary arch generate an as yet uncharacterised molecule that attracts sensory fibres of the maxillary ganglion of the mouse. They do so only at a particular time in development (embryonic day 10) and the maxillary axons themselves are only susceptible to it at the same time. In the animal the attractant probably serves to draw the sensory fibres into the epithelium as they are passing by rather than to direct the initial direction of outgrowth from the ganglion. Similar transient local attraction may explain the late development of sprouting side branches from axons whose main growth cones have previously passed by a nucleus on the way to a second destination (O'Leary & Terashima, 1988). Another role of chemotropism might be to direct the initial outgrowth of axons. Tessier-Lavigne *et al.* (1988) have shown *in vitro* that the floor plate cells of the developing spinal cord can attract axons of commissural afferents, which *in vivo* have to grow from the dorsal into the ventral horn of the spinal cord before crossing the midline.

Schwann cells have also been suggested as part of a guidance mechanism in the mammalian peripheral nervous system, whereby the Schwann cells are the pathfinders and axons follow their attractive lead (see Keynes, 1987). Harrison (1908) showed that removal of Schwann cells by ablation of the neural crest did not stop amphibian motor nerves finding their correct muscles and in chick limbs Schwann cells appear to lag behind the incoming axons (Dahm & Landmesser, 1988). On the other hand others claim that Schwann cells enter the chick limb before axons and that their removal impedes axon ingrowth (Noakes & Bennett, 1987; Noakes, Bennett & Stratford, 1988). As derivatives of the neural crest, Schwann cells would not be expected to correct their migration trajectories when transplanted to abnormal sites (see Chapter 3); moreover, Landmesser's observations of pathway correction in the chick limb (see below) are not consistent with a direction finding role of Schwann cells. It is therefore likely that they provide only trophic but not tropic support to the axons.

Cell surface and extracellular matrix molecules

Immunological methods have led to the discovery and isolation of many molecules that may play a part in neuronal cell adhesion and migration (Chapter 4) and axonal growth (Chapter 5). At present no consensus has emerged about the precise roles of the various molecules (all seem to have several functions) or their relative importance or even about their names, as different groups of workers using a variety of animal species have frequently discovered or rediscovered already known molecules. There is no ideal classification (see Lander, 1989). A simple catalogue for vertebrate species is given in Table 6.1 and a summary of the location and proposed functions is given in Table 6.2. A diagram of possible roles is given in

Table 6.1. *Molecules involved in cell migration and axon growth*

Name	Similar or identical molecules	Ligand	Comments
Cell surface molecules			
N-cadherin (mouse)	N-CalCAM (chick) A-CAM (chick)	N-cadherin (homophilic)	Adhesion needs calcium ions
N-CAM	BSP-2	N-CAM (homophilic)	Also found in muscle. Adhesion calcium-independent. HNK1 carbohydrate epitope
L1 (mouse)	NILE[a] (rat) G4, Ng-CAM, 8D9 (chick)	L1 (homophilic)	Located on axons. HNK1 carbohydrate epitope
TAG-1 (rat)	—	?	Transiently expressed on only certain parts of axons
Integrin complex	CSAT[b] antigen (chick)	Laminin Fibronectin Molecules with RGD sequence	May also react with N-CAM
AMOG[c]	—	?	
Extracellular matrix molecules			
Laminin	—	Integrin	RGD sequence may be involved + others
Fibronectin	—	Integrin	RGD sequence involved
Tenascin	Cytotactin, J1, myotendinous antigen	?	HNK1 epitope

Note:
[a] Nerve growth factor Inducible Large External Glycoprotein.
[b] Cell Substratum Attachment AnTibody.
[c] Adhesion Molecule On Glia.

Table 6.2. *Location and roles of cell surface and extracellular matrix molecules*

Name	Locations	Possible roles			
		Tissue formation and cell adhesion	Neuron migration	Axon fasciculation	Axon growth
N-cadherin	Neural ectoderm. Nervous system generally. More on sensory than motor axons. Muscle. Embryonic mesoderm.	+	−	+	+
N-CAM	Neural ectoderm and nervous system. Glia (less than on neurons). Embryonic muscle. Adult muscle endplate. Denervated adult muscle. Embryonic mesoderm.	+	−	+	+
L1	Axons. Schwann cells and glia.	−	−	+	+
Integrins	Widely spread on many cell types.	−	+	−	+
AMOG	Astrocytes, oligodendrocytes.	−	+	−	−
Laminin	Basal Laminae and other extracellular locations within and outside CNS.	−	+	−	+
Fibronectin	Many sites outside CNS. Restricted sites in CNS.	−	+	−	+
Tenascin	Glia, fibroblasts, somites, denervated muscle, developing CNS.	−	−	−	+

Homophilic cell-cell interactions

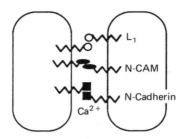

Growth on cell surface

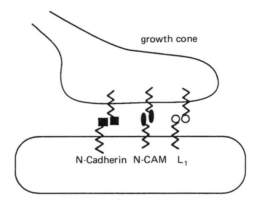

Growth on extracellular matrix

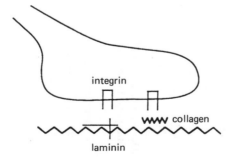

Fig. 6.3. Diagram of location and possible function of some cell adhesion and extracellular matrix molecules.

fig. 6.3. Three further glycoproteins (fasciclins I,II and III) involved in axon guidance in insects are discussed briefly on p.66.

The obvious distinction made in the tables and diagram between cell-attached surface molecules and extracellular matrix molecules is not sacrosanct, as N-CAM and L1 also occur in secreted forms in the extracellular matrix (Cole & Glaser, 1986; Booth & Brown, 1988; Sweadner, 1983). Furthermore, attachment molecules may have additional properties; for example, part of the laminin molecule has a distinct domain with growth factor activity (Panayatou *et al.*, 1989). There appears to be much duplication in function amongst those molecules that have been found; for example antibodies to several molecules (N-CAM, N-cadherin and integrin) may be needed simultaneously to block axon growth completely in some situations (Bixby *et al.*, 1987). Mechanisms underlying the function of cell surface and extracellular matrix molecules are as yet unclear. When cell–cell or cell–extracellular matrix interactions cause changes in gene expression or whole cell movement, some form of second messenger will be needed as an intermediary, but axonal growth or cell aggregation could be encouraged simply by providing mechanical adhesion.

N-Cadherin is an integral membrane glycoprotein that needs Ca^{2+} ions if it is to promote intercellular adhesion. It is part of a family of cadherins (Takeichi, 1988). The timing of its appearance and disappearance during development suggests that this molecule is involved mainly in cell sorting and in holding together cells in a tissue; it is present on neural crest cells before and after, but not during migration (Hatta *et al.* 1987). Furthermore, antibodies to cadherins cause tissue disruption (Duband *et al.*, 1987). A change in the type of cadherin expressed in ectodermal cells on the neural plate from E (epithelial) to N (neural) may help to account for the formation of the neural tube (see Jessell, 1988). In addition N-cadherin may also be important in helping axons to grow on other axons and on astrocytes (Tomaselli *et al.*, 1988).

N-CAM (Neural Cell Adhesion Molecule) is present on most neurons and in embryonic and denervated adult skeletal muscle. It is also present at the normal adult neuromuscular junction. The extracellular domain of N-CAM has repeated segments that have structural similarities to the variable region of immunoglobulins. N-CAM comes in various forms with differing molecular weights and membrane attachments and there are differences between neural and muscle N-CAM. The degree of glycosylation also varies, there being both high (H) (embryonic) and low (L) (adult) carbohydrate-containing variants. Like N-cadherin it may function as a general 'glue' for cells, for its expression falls when neural crest cells migrate and rises when they stop (see Jessell, 1988). However N-CAM is also likely to be important as a general facilitator of axon growth and for encouraging axons to grow together (fasciculate). For example, ingrowth of motor axons to muscle coincides with the appearance of N-CAM on the muscle fibres (Tosney *et al.*, 1986) and antibodies to N-CAM disrupt motor axon growth on myotubes in culture (Rutishauser, Grumet & Edelman, 1983) and reduce sprouting of motor axons in paralysed muscles (Booth, Kemplay & Brown, 1990) and also disrupt the fasciculation of optic axons growing into the tectum (Thanos *et al.*, 1984). The relative proportions of N-CAM and L1 expressed on muscle and motor axons may determine the pattern of axon branching in chick muscle (Landmesser *et al.*, 1988). N-CAM adhesion may also trigger production of choline acetyltransferase in embryonic chick sympathetic neurons (Acheson & Rutishauser, 1988).

L1, like N-CAM, also belongs to the immunoglobulin gene superfamily; interestingly, the family includes other molecules involved in cell–cell recognition such as the MHC antigens and immunoglobulin receptors (Williams, 1985). L1 binds homophilically to other L1 molecules. It is present on some axons and may even be localised to parts of axons. Antibodies to it prevent fasciculation and slow axonal growth (Chang, Rathjen & Raper, 1987). Another molecule capable of mediating neuron–glia adhesion and neuron–neuron adhesion also has structural similarities in its extracellular portion to immunoglobulin constant region domains. It is called Myelin Associated Glycoprotein (MAG) (see review by Lander, 1989).

TAG-1 has a less widespread and more transient expression than L1 and so its appearance may help to alter axon growth at particular points on their course. In the spinal cord TAG-1 is expressed on commissural axons that project from the dorsal horn to the ventral part of the cord and across the midline floorplate. Thereafter the axons are devoid of TAG-1 and express L1 as they proceed to run longitudinally in the white matter (Dodd & Jessell, 1988). The change in expression may be mediated by interaction with cells of the floor plate.

Integrins are integral membrane proteins composed of non-covalently linked α and β chains. Both the α and β chains can vary in their detailed structures making it possible for different integrins to be more or less attractive to different molecules in the extracellular matrix, for which they are the main cell-attached ligand. Both fibronection and laminin may be recognised by integrins because they possess a tripeptide group composed of Arg–Gly–Asp (RGD sequence); laminin is also recognised by nerve cells at a second site near the end of its long arm (see reviews by Jessell, 1988, and Edgar, 1989). Antibodies against integrins inhibit extension of axons on laminin (Tomaselli *et al.*, 1988). Nerve cells could change their affinity for substrates like laminin by changing the precise structure of their integrins. The integrins could remain useful for axon interaction with other molecules, for some can interact with adhesion molecules such as N-CAM and L1, which possess immunoglobulin-like domains (Marlin & Springer, 1987).

Laminin is a cross-shaped molecule made up from three polypeptide chains (Paulsson *et al.*, 1985) and may link to integrins via an RGD sequence (Hynes, 1987). Interference with the interaction of neural crest cells with laminin by using antibodies to laminin or integrins, or by using RGD peptides, perturbs their migration in chick embryos (see Jessell, 1988). Laminin *in vitro* is an excellent substrate for some types of axonal growth (Carbonetto *et al.*, 1987), and is present in appropriate places *in vivo*, both in the peripheral nervous system (e.g. the basal lamina of Schwann cells; Cornbrooks *et al.*, 1983) and in the CNS (e.g. where axons grow across the developing corpus callosum; Liesi & Silver, 1988).

Other molecules that may be involved in nerve cell migration and axonal extension include collagens, proteoglycans and oligosaccharides (Rutishauser & Jessell, 1988). Association with proteoglycans may be important for optimal functioning of both laminin (Chiu, Matthew & Patterson, 1986) and N-CAM (Cole & Glaser, 1986).

Target recognition

When axons arrive in the general vicinity of their target, they have to 'recognise' or make long-lasting contacts with the correct target cells so that specialised contacts between axon and target can then develop. This means recognising not only the correct type of cell ('type' specificity), but in many cases also a small subset of these cells, defined by their position in the target ('place' specificity).

Type specificity

This is readily demonstrated in tissue culture using time-lapse photography: sympathetic nerves, for example, will form long-lasting contacts with smooth muscle cells but not fibroblasts (Burnstock, 1981). Many cross-innervation experiments *in vivo* have also been performed to investigate type specificity. Early experiments showed that functional synaptic contacts were not established between grossly mismatched axons and targets, such as sensory nerves and muscles (Gutmann, 1945). However, if the axon releases the appropriate transmitter, synapses can form, but with variable success (Landmesser, 1971, 1972; Purves, 1976; Ostberg *et al.*, 1976; Sayers & Tonge, 1982). Similar experiments have been performed more recently to investigate the specificity of neurons for CNS targets. When five different types of foetal cholinergic graft were made into the hippocampus of adult rats, in which the normal septal innervation had been destroyed, the most successful innervation was made by transplanted septal neurons themselves (Nilssen *et al.*, 1988).

Place specificity

There is now abundant evidence that cells of similar type within some target tissues are labelled according to their position. A striking demonstration of this was provided by the cross-innervation experiments of Wigston & Sanes (1982, 1985), who found that intercostal muscles taken from different rib spaces in rats were reinnervated more intensively by cholinergic sympathetic axons originating from the same segmental level. Several lines of evidence also suggest place-specific labels on axons and muscle fibres within a single muscle: during postnatal development in rats there is a selective withdrawal of motor axon branches from muscle fibres in a manner that enhances the topographical projection from the motor pool to the muscle (Brown & Booth, 1983); a similar projection is reestablished following reinnervation in the neonate or adult (Hardman & Brown, 1987; Laskowski & Sanes, 1988); finally, motor axons that have reinnervated incorrect muscles are displaced when correct axons return, at least in amphibia (Dennis & Yip, 1978).

Place-specific labelling of neurons in the CNS is the most likely explanation for the observations on the innervation of the retina of fish and amphibia. Axons arising from different parts of the retina have a propensity to make synapses in particular parts of the optic tectum, even if the route taken to the tectum is abnormal (Fujisawa, 1981) or the tectal cells are moved (Hope, Hammond & Gaze, 1976). If only part of the retina is available to innervate the developing tectum, the axons of the remaining retinal ganglion cells still synapse in the right place and do not take the opportunity of innervating other sites now available to them (Holt, 1984). The demonstration that cells isolated from different parts of the retina adhere preferentially to their corresponding area of the tectum (Barbera, Marchase & Roth, 1973) provided direct evidence for place-specific affinities between axons and targets in this system.

The use of monoclonal antibodies is the most likely avenue for isolation and characterisation of the cell surface molecules responsible for place specificity. Monoclonal antibodies have now been isolated that can differentiate different parts of the retina (Trisler, Schneider & Nirenberg, 1981), the tectum (Trisler & Collins, 1987), chick limb buds (Ohsugi & Ide, 1986) and even the whole rostro-caudal axis of the rat nervous system (Suzue, Imrick & Patterson, 1988).

Specific vertebrate systems

Innervation of limbs

In the 1930s, observations on the reinnervation of denervated or transplanted limbs in tailed amphibians led to the erroneous belief that specific guidance and recognition played only a minimal part in the establishment of connections between peripheral nerves and their targets. It was found that nerves regenerated into the limbs in a profuse and apparently disordered manner, and yet normal movements and reflexes were soon established. It was therefore reasoned that muscles and sensory end-organs in the limb were innervated at random, but were able to confer identity on their nerves to permit appropriate reorganisation of central connections (the theory of 'myotypic specification'). A similar conclusion was drawn from the misdirected 'wiping' reflexes seen in adult frogs in which a piece of belly skin had been transplanted onto the back and a piece of back skin onto the belly when the animal was a tadpole (Miner, 1956). More recent work has shown that regenerating motor and sensory axons in salamanders and axolotls grow through the limb tissues until they find their correct muscles, even if the nerves are deliberately misdirected (Grimm, 1971; Wilson, Tonge & Holder, 1989; Heidemann, 1977). Where misdirected axons are rigorously prevented from reaching their correct muscles, uncoordinated movements persist indefinitely (Mark, 1965). These experiments demonstrated the existence of mechanisms that can accomplish accurate reinnervation in some lower vertebrates, apparently by target recognition as the regenerating axons ramify through the tissues. In adult mammals the axons remain confined to the muscles they are guided to by the nerve trunks, and reinnervation following nerve section does not reestablish correct connectons. Neonatal mammals show some of the specificity of amphibia (Gerding, Robbins & Antosiak, 1977; Aldskogius & Thomander, 1986).

None of these experiments sheds any real light on the mechanisms that connect axons with their targets in the developing limb. As always, advances came with the introduction of a new technique, in this case the labelling of axons in the developing limb with horseradish peroxidase (HRP). In the first experiments HRP injected into the developing muscles of *Xenopus* tadpoles revealed that some are innervated by motoneurons in regions of the spinal cord that do not innervate these muscles in the adult, implying imprecise guidance mechanisms. The erroneous projections were thought to be removed by neuronal death (Lamb, 1977). Later work using bullfrog tadpoles found a precise motor neuron projection pattern at all stages (Farel & Bemelmans, 1985), raising the possibility that the earlier results arose from spread of labelling material between muscles.

The HRP labelling technique has also revealed very accurate guidance of motor axons to the limb muscles of chick embryos (Landmesser, 1978). The motor axons have been found to project in a highly ordered fashion to the muscle masses from which the muscles develop: medial motor neurons project to the ventral muscle mass, lateral motor neurons to the dorsal mass, and the rostro-caudal position of neurons correlates with the axon terminations in the anterior–posterior axis of each muscle mass. This orderly arrangement could be achieved in principle by passive channelling, although it is difficult to imagine how the axons from the cell bodies of a future pool would come together passively from different spinal roots. Alternatively the identity of each pool could be specified in the cord and connections established by active guidance.

The experiments designed to determine which of these mechanisms operates in the establishment of muscle innervation in chick limbs rely on observing the pattern of connections that develops when motor neurons or limbs have been translocated or partly deleted. In the most elegant of these

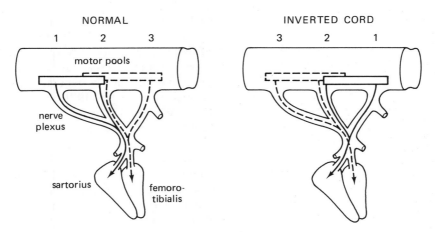

Fig. 6.4. Pathways taken by axons from motoneuron pools for two muscles in the normal chick embryo (left). After inversion of the spinal cord, axons are still guided to their correct muscle (right).

experiments (Lance-Jones & Landmesser, 1980) a length of the neural tube consisting of 3–4 segments in the lumbosacral region was reversed in the cranio-caudal direction (fig. 6.4). At later stages the reversed motor neurons and the pathways of their axons were labelled following HRP injection into the muscles. The neurons were found to have formed their original pools and functional connections in spite of the anterior–posterior shifts in their position and entry points into the nerve plexus. Moreover HRP injected into specific reversed cord segments before axons had reached the muscle masses labelled the outgrowing axons in the nerve plexus and showed that they made specific alterations to their pathways to reach their appropriate muscle nerves. These observations imply that axons actively select the pathways to their own muscles by responding to local cues encountered as they grow between spinal cord and muscles. It has been possible to confirm this active selection by directly observing the growth cones of motor axons in live Zebra fish using either Nomarski optics or by labelling the neurons with fluorescent dyes (Myers, Eisen & Westerfield, 1986). The growing axon from each motor neuron follows a stereotyped pathway which is unique for different types of motor neuron. This involves changes in direction of growth at particular places. No mistakes of projection seem to be made.

The guidance cues are able to compensate for cord reversals and limb shifts over several segments, but axons cannot make pathway corrections for larger displacements (Lance-Jones & Landmesser, 1982) or distal limb rotations (Summerbell & Stirling, 1981). Under these circumstances non-specific cues appear to channel axons to the wrong muscles. In supernumerary limbs axons from inappropriate levels may still respond to the guidance cues in some patterned way to produce an apparent 'hierarchy of specificities' (Hollyday, 1981), but the fact that the wrong muscles are successfully innervated in these experiments is evidence that target recognition appears to play a minor role in setting up the initial pattern of innervation of muscles in chicks. This seems to be borne out by the fact that the major axon pathways in the limb can form in the complete absence of muscle following focal X-irradiation of somites in early embryos (Lewis *et al.*, 1981). Yet under these conditions individual muscle nerves do not form. Furthermore, in normal circumstances the correct groups of motor axons must leave the main nerves at the right place so that they and they alone grow into a particular muscle. Hence some form of guidance or recognition mechanism must operate close to the target muscle to allow correct choices to be made in the normal intact system and to allow alternative choices when conditions are perturbed. Perhaps muscle fibres generate a chemotactic factor that attracts motor axons non-specifically while the connective tissue contains markers that contain more specific information (Wigston & Donahue, 1988; Lance-Jones, 1988). The connective tissue and tendons of muscle are derived from local mesenchymal cells, but myofibres develop from precursor cells that migrate into the limb from the somitic myotome (Chevalier, Kieny & Mauger, 1977). Although each limb muscle receives precursor cells from only a limited and reproducible number of somites (Beresford, 1983), the specific cues appear to be unrelated to the somitic origin of the muscles, because rotations of the embryonic myotome, which lead to altered segmental populations of muscle precursor cells in the developing muscles, do not change their innervation (Keynes *et al.*, 1987). In keeping with the presence of local guidance cues, motor axons wait outside developing muscles before growing in, a behaviour which is reminiscent of the marked slowing of growth at the plexus choice points (Dahm & Landmesser, 1988).

Once within muscle, the branching patterns of axons may be determined by the relative adhesiveness of axons to each other and to the muscle fibres (Landmesser *et al.*, 1988). Adhesiveness to the muscle fibres appears to be related to the amount of N-CAM on their surfaces, which is reduced by activity (Covault & Sanes, 1985). This would provide a simple but effective means for establishing complete innervation.

The sensory innervation of chick limbs has also been investigated with the same techniques that have been applied to the motor system. In the normal animal the initial pattern of pathways of sensory axons from the ganglia at various segmental levels is found to be the same as in the adult (Honig, 1982; Scott, 1982), suggesting the existence of an active guidance mechanism. However sensory axons seem to lag behind motor axons as they enter the limb and their growth cones never become flattened and enlarged (Tosney & Landmesser, 1985). When motor axons are prevented from entering the limb no sensory axons enter the muscles (Swanson & Lewis, 1986). Muscle sensory fibres therefore seem to depend on motor axons for guidance. Moreover the sensory axons are not particular about which motor axons to follow, for if the sensory ganglia are displaced by rotation of the neural crest, sensory axons follow the first motor axons they encounter rather than seeking out those that correspond to their original segmental level (Scott, 1987). It appears that guidance of sensory axons is less rigidly specified than guidance of motor axons.

Projection of retina to tectum

The majority of fibre tracts in the CNS connect cells in one region to cells in another in a smooth, topologically continuous manner. The establishment of this order has been studied extensively in the projection of the retinal ganglion cells from the eye to the tectum, the main visual processing centre in non-mammalian vertebrates. Experiments on adult amphibians initiated by Sperry in the 1940s indicated that target recognition might be important in the development of the retinotectal projection. Using a behavioural assay, Sperry found that normal vision was eventually restored if the optic nerve was cut, but that inverted vision developed if the eye had also been rotated (Sperry, 1943). Sperry's explanation was that retinal and tectal cells are in some way labelled and reestablish their original connections on the tectum by 'chemoaffinity' (Sperry, 1963); rotation of the eye apparently had no effect on this reconnection process, so when vision was restored the animal 'saw' the world upside down and behaved accordingly.

The chemoaffinity hypothesis has since been substantiated by several lines of evidence. First, regenerating axons are disordered in the optic nerve (Fujisawa, 1981), are very widespread in their initial distribution on the tectum (Meyer, 1980), but ultimately terminate only in appropriate circumscribed tectal locations. There is recent evidence that some degree of order is restored in the optic nerve such that axons from similar sectors of the retina become reassociated as they grow (Bernhardt & Easter, 1988), but regenerating axons are clearly not guided straight to their original sites. Secondly, the appropriate regenerating retinal axons will make correct connections with a piece of rotated or translocated tectum (e.g. Hope *et al.*, 1976). This implies that the restoration of a correctly oriented projection cannot just be due to ordering of retinal axons amongst themselves on the tectal surface. Thirdly, Walter *et al.* (1987) found that fibres of ganglion cells from the temporal part of the retina grew best on membranes derived from the anterior part of the tectum, which is the part of the tectum where they normally make synapses. They could also grow on membranes from posterior tectum but given a choice (a series of alternating stripes of anterior and posterior derived membranes) their axons all grew along the strips coated with anterior-derived membranes. Fourthly, it has been shown in reinnervation experiments in the goldfish (Meyer, 1984, 1987;

Hayes & Meyer, 1988) that optic axons can discriminate between lateral and medial tectum even in adult fish after long periods of tectal denervation showing that in this species stable labels persist. Although inappropriate connections can be made, the synaptic density in correct locations is greater.

The chemoaffinity hypothesis requires elaboration to make it consistent with observations of another phenomenon in the retino-tectal system, that of repositioning of retinal ganglion cell terminals on the tectum. Repositioning has to occur gradually during normal development because new retinal ganglion cells, which are added uniformly around the perimeter of the retina, project uniformly to the perimeter of the tectum, which grows only at its caudal margin (Gaze *et al.*, 1979). This repositioning of the retinal axons' synaptic sites can be recognised in the characteristic shapes of the arbours of the optic axons in the adult tectum (Schmidt, 1984). Repositioning also occurs when half retinae innervate whole tecta, or whole retinae innervate half tecta: although discontinuous projections predicted by a rigid chemoaffinity hypothesis are reestablished initially, these are gradually expanded or compressed until there is a continuous and uniform projection from retina to tectum (Gaze, 1974). To accommodate these observations it has been suggested that the affinities between axons and tectal cells are graded, and that axon terminals compete with each other for the occupancy of limited sites on tectal cells. Computer models based on this idea can reproduce the phenomena described above (e.g. Whitelaw & Cowan, 1981).

The above discussion relates predominantly to the organisation of afferents on the tectal surface. There is good evidence that during development optic axons are actively guided on their way to the tectum and that this helps to simplify the task of achieving order in the tectum. The axons from the retinal ganglion cells traverse the retina radially to the optic nerve head, and then travel down the optic nerve in a more or less orderly array (Fawcett, 1981). However, as the fibres travel through the optic tract on the surface of the diencephalon, this ordering is lost as fibres interweave amongst one another to establish a new order such that axons are delivered directly to their appropriate sites on the tectum. The reordering is demonstrated elegantly in the ribbon-shaped optic nerve and optic tract of cichlid fish (Scholes, 1979). It now seems clear that active guidance in the optic tract is responsible for this reorganisation, because the fibres that first grow out from both halves of a compound eye (produced experimentally by replacing one retinal half by its opposite half from another eye) are delivered to the same parts of the tectum via the same branches of the tract that they would normally occupy (Straznicky, Gaze & Keating, 1981).

Finally, technical advances have now made it possible to observe *in vivo* the ingrowth of optic axons in developing *Xenopus* (Harris *et al.*, 1987). The results support the deductions made about guidance and recognition in other experiments on developing and regenerating systems. Retinal axons are seen to grow straight towards the tectum, slow on nearing it, when their growth cones get more complex (behaviour reminiscent of motor axons at choice points) then choose correct termination sites even when alternatives have been made available experimentally (Holt, 1984). Thus, as in the limb, axons are guided in the correct direction, make active decisions along the pathway and eventually use place-specific target labelling to sort out their final relative positions.

An intriguing problem in guidance in the CNS is exemplified in the retinotectal projection at the optic chiasm. Here the bundles of axons of identical type and function from each eye pass through each other (decussate) as they run to their contralateral termination sites. Many similar projections occur throughout the sensory and motor systems. The simplest explanation for the phenomenon of decussation is that axons tend to grow in straight lines, and because they converge at approximately 90° in the region of decussation they cross into the contralateral pathway. However, this explanation appears to be inadequate at the chiasm of animals with forward facing eyes and hence a large area of binocular overlap in the visual field: here axons from the nasal half of the retina decussate, but the temporal fibres remain ipsilateral, presumably to allow images of an object seen in both eyes to be processed together in higher visual areas on one side of the brain. Recent work shows that the position of ipsilaterally projecting axons in the optic nerve of rats is not confined to a particular region of the nerve, which implies that a passive guidance mechanism is unlikely to be enough to account for their choice of the ipsilateral optic tract (Jeffery, 1989). Whatever active guidance mechanisms are responsible for partial decussation at the chiasm, they may be imperfect, because initially many axons take mistaken routes towards the inappropriate side of the brain (Land & Lund, 1979) or even towards the other eye (Bunt & Lund, 1981). Some of these aberrant axons are removed by cell death. Curiously, decussation of the optic nerves in adult albino animals is more complete than in normal adults, and the pigmented cells which albinos lack appear to be important in guiding the retinal axons in the optic nerve (Silver & Sapiro, 1981). However, there are no gross differences between albino and normal rats in the initial retino-collicular projections (Land & Lund, 1979), so the role of pigmented cells in guidance is still unclear.

Innervation of sympathetic ganglia

In 1897 Langley reported that a cut preganglionic nerve regenerated into the superior cervical ganglion and that normal function was restored to the sympathetic end-organs. He suggested that a selective reinnervation of ganglion cells had occurred, brought about by a chemical matching of pre- and post-ganglionic neurons with the same function. Recent study of this phenomenon of target recognition has shown that ganglion cells are innervated and reinnervated preferentially by preganglionic axons that arise from 3–4 contiguous segmental levels of the cord (Njå & Purves, 1977*a,b*). Segmental specificity is also displayed in the reinnervation of thoracic and lumbar ganglia transplanted in place of the superior cervical ganglion: cells in the transplanted ganglia are innervated more effectively by axons in the preganglionic trunk arising from more caudal spinal nerves (Purves, Thompson & Yip, 1981). Graded affinities and competition also modulate the chemoaffinity between preganglionic axons and ganglion cells, because the pattern of connections depends on the number and composition of the axons that are competing as well as the number and composition of the target cells (Leistol, Maehlen & Njå, 1986).

As preganglionic sympathetic axons from various segmental levels show a tendency to innervate *intercostal muscles* from their own thoracic levels (Wigston & Sanes, 1982, 1985) it seems that graded segmental labels common to a variety of tissues may exist. In the superior cervical ganglion in particular it appears that different cells carry different segmental labels (Njå & Purves, 1977*a*), probably in addition to function-specific labels. The labels might be induced retrogradely on the cell bodies when the axons of the cells first contact the various target organs, which would be a logical extension of the hypothesis that transmitter phenotypes of crest cells are specified by local environmental influences (see Chapter 3). If this is so, then the induced labels must become permanent in the adult, because they are not respecified when the postganglionic axons regenerate to different target organs (Purves & Thompson, 1979). It is more likely, however, that the labels exist on the ganglion cells before pre- and post-synaptic innervation occurs (Rubin, 1985). The labels would then be responsible for establishing the specificity of presynaptic connections by a mechanism of target recognition. Such labels would be unlikely to be conferred by spatial gradients in the ganglion, because ganglion cells that innervate particular target organs are scattered throughout the ganglion (Lichtman, Purves & Yip, 1979). The labels would therefore probably be specified before the cells migrate to the ganglion.

Pathfinding in the central and peripheral nervous systems of insects

In insects a scaffolding of glial cells is laid out early on in the developing CNS and provides a framework for both commissural and longitudinally running nerve fibres (Jacobs & Goodman, 1989). Axons are guided along this framework by contact with the glial cells or basement membrane and later arriving axons are also guided by the axons already in place.

Unlike axons in vertebrates some of those in the CNS of insects appear to be rigidly 'chemo-specified' in that they are unable to grow at all if the other neurons on whose axons they specifically fasciculate are removed

(Bastiani *et al.*, 1985). There seems to be no possibility of gaining the correct target by an abnormal route. As axons navigate along their chosen partner the filopodia of their growth cones can invaginate deeply into the membrane of the other cell and at decision points where changes of direction are made the growth cone can take on a more complex appearance (Bastiani *et al.*, 1985).

Attempts are now underway to study the molecular basis of chemospecificity both in grasshoppers (Bastiani *et al.*, 1987) and fruit flies (Patel, Snow & Goodman, 1987) using monoclonal antibodies raised against developing ganglia. Three glycoproteins (fasciclins I, II and III) have been found which are expressed only on subsets of neurons during the time of axon outgrowth and which therefore might be involved in specific axon guidance. Interestingly, the gene for fasciclin II is a member of the immunoglobulin gene superfamily and fasciclin II has structural similarities to N-CAM. It is expressed particularly on some longitudinally running axons. Antibodies to it can perturb their growth (Harrelson & Goodman, 1988).

Guidance of sensory axons in insects, which arise from cells in the periphery, seems to be somewhat different from guidance of axons in the CNS for a variety of cues seem to be available. Neither the presence of other axons arising earlier in development nor regions of low cell density seem to be essential (Blair & Palka, 1985) and it has been proposed that the cells over which the axons grow are polarised to provide directionality (Berlot & Goodman, 1984). At entry into the CNS, however, the presence of the correct specific guide post cell is needed if the ingrowing axon is not to remain marooned in the developing appendage (Palka, 1986).

So accurate is the guidance in many insect pathways that positional signals on the target might appear at first sight unnecessary. However, where several sensory axons converge on the neuropil and each carries specific spatial information, a degree of organisation in the terminal sites is needed if the information is not to be lost. Such place-specific choice is seen in the projection from the wind detecting hair cells of the cercal system in crickets (Murphey, 1985). If hair cells are transplanted from one cercus to a different position, the sensory neuron that is transplanted with them regrows its axon and this terminates in its correct original location in the neuropil. There is evidence that the sensory cell gains its knowledge of where to grow from its position in the cercus at the time it arises from its precursor during development.

Chapter 7

Development of axon–target and axon–glial cell contacts

Synaptogenesis

Introduction
Synapse formation requires the incoming axon to change from a state of growth to that appropriate for release of transmitter from a stationary terminal. In the postsynaptic cell, changes appropriate for receiving transmitter occur in the region of membrane destined to become the junction, and extrajunctional membrane properties also change. These changes are accompanied by the development of structural specialisations in the pre- and post-synaptic cells.

Formation of the neuromuscular junction
The neuromuscular junction has been subjected to more experimentation than other synapses in attempts to identify and characterise each step in the process of synaptogenesis. The major contributions have come from three sorts of experiment: regeneration of synapses in adults when a nerve grows back to its original synaptic sites; synapse formation at new sites on denervated adult muscle fibres; and formation of synapses between embryonic nerve and muscle cells in tissue culture. In addition, application of the techniques of patch clamp and molecular biology have shed new light on the development of specific junctional transmitter receptor molecules.

The halting of axon extension and the start of chemical transmission are the first steps in synapse formation. The muscle must also instruct the nerve to develop specialised release sites and almost certainly supplies some form of survival or growth factor to the motor axons (see Chapter 8). The motor axons cause aggregation of pre-existing acetylcholine receptors at the synapse and initiate production of synapse-specific acetylcholine receptors and synapse-specific molecules for the basal lamina. They also cause the eventual disappearance of acetylcholine receptors outside the region of the new junction by suppressing their production, prevent further innervation of muscle fibres and stimulate the production of junctional folds in the postsynaptic membrane. These steps are summarised in fig. 7.1.

It seems likely that specific postsynaptic surface molecules are needed for

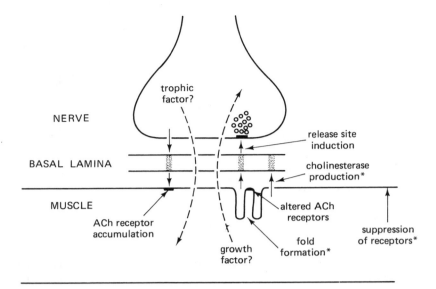

Fig. 7.1. Development of the neuromuscular juction. Events marked with an asterisk (*) need postsynaptic activity. ACh = acetylcholine.

a synapse to form (Chapter 6). These molecules are at first widely distributed, for in denervated adult muscles ectopic junctions can be formed at many sites along a muscle fibre's length (Lømo, 1980). The normal position of junctions in the middle of the long axis of muscle fibres is probably not due to any initial specialisation at that point but to the short length of myotubes when first contacted, followed by growth at each end of the fibre. Once an initial site is formed, however, several motor axons converge on it, leading to a phase of multiple innervation (see Chapter 9 and fig. 7.2). In adult muscles too, original synaptic sites are preferentially innervated by axons returning to a denervated muscle (Bennett, McClachlan & Taylor, 1973).

The subcellular mechanisms that bring axon growth to a halt are not known. Observations on adult frog muscles killed by freezing showed that regenerating motor axons stopped growing and formed normal presynaptic specialisations when they regenerated onto the basal lamina of the old neuromuscular junctions, even in the complete absence of muscle cells (Sanes, Marshall & McMahan, 1978). This suggests strongly that axon growth inhibition and presynaptic differentiation are under the control of some substance in the basal lamina. During development similar or identical substances may be present in the muscle membrane and inhibit axon growth when the axons first contact it. A synapse-specific form of laminin has been identified that might act as the stop signal for arriving

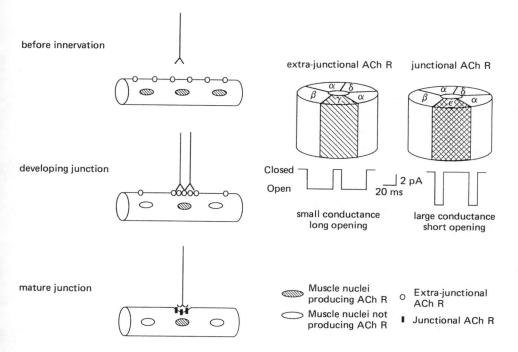

Fig. 7.2. Changes in acetylcholine receptor (AChR) distribution, composition and physiological properties at developing neuromuscular junctions.

motor axons (Hunter *et al.*, 1989). Recent experiments in a different system (the visual pathway) have demonstrated that retinal ganglion cells down-regulate their laminin receptors on contact with their target cells in the optic tectum (Cohen *et al.*, 1989) and this could be a mechanism that might bring axonal advance to a halt. Another possibility is that specific recognition molecules trigger capping of microtubules and neurofilaments (Mitchison & Kirschner, 1988) so that transported precursors are no longer incorporated but shipped back to the cell body (Hollenbeck & Bray, 1987).

A rudimentary form of synaptic transmission is established from the moment motor axons make contact with muscle fibres (Chow & Poo, 1985), because transmitter released from the growth cones activates acetylcholine receptors that are distributed in clusters throughout the muscle fibre surface (Diamond & Miledi, 1962). As the terminal matures transmitter is released by exocytosis at specialised active zones, which in the neuromuscular junction are in register with the clefts between the tops of the secondary folds of the postsynaptic membrane. These release sites also can form in the presence of only the synaptic basal lamina (Glicksman & Sanes, 1983) and their formation during development is presumably also mediated by contact with some substance on the muscle fibre surface. Transmitter release and other aspects of the development of the presynaptic terminal may also be influenced by growth factors released by the muscle. Certainly motor neuron survival depends upon early contact with muscle during development (see Chapter 8) and in other neurons, e.g. sympathetic ganglion cells, uptake of Nerve Growth Factor can change transmitter output by increasing production of transmitter synthesising enzymes (Thoenen *et al.*, 1971; Lindsay & Harman, 1989).

The accumulation of transmitter receptors at the neuromuscular junction, which occurs initially by lateral migration of receptors from surrounding muscle areas (Anderson & Cohen, 1977), is the first major postsynaptic event in synaptogenesis. There is now strong evidence that this is caused by a substance liberated from or attached to nerve terminals. First, if both nerve and muscle cells are killed, a chemical marker that is left behind in the junctional basal lamina can induce receptor accumulation in myotubes regenerating within the intact lamina (Burden, Sargent & McMahon, 1979). Secondly, even degenerating nerves that have made only brief contact with muscle prior to axotomy leave behind a marker that stimulates receptor accumulation at extrajunctional sites on denervated muscle (Lømo & Slater, 1980*a*). Thirdly, a factor named 'agrin' isolated from the electric organ of *Torpedo californica*, increases receptor aggregation on cultured muscle cells (Smith *et al.*, 1987) and is present in the basal lamina at the neuromuscular junction and in motor neurons (Magill-Salc & McMahan, 1988). Agrin appears to be specific to motor axons, as neither sensory nor sympathetic nerves will induce aggregation of acetylcholine receptors on muscle cells in culture (Cohen & Weldon, 1980). (It is, however, possible to cause acetylcholine receptor accumulation on amphibian myocytes in culture with positively charged latex beads (Peng & Cheng, 1982).) It is implicit in these findings that receptor accumulation occurs in the absence of electrical activity, and this has been confirmed for synapse development *in vivo* and *in vitro* (e.g. Cohen, 1972). A receptor associated protein (RAPsyn) is probably involved in stabilising the receptors at the junction, but its expression is not regulated by innervation (Frail *et al.*, 1989), unlike the acetylcholine receptors (see below).

The subsequent postsynaptic events in neuromuscular synaptogenesis include, in the approximate order of their occurrence: accumulation of acetylcholinesterase and other molecules in the basal lamina at the junction; loss of the ability of non-innervated membrane to accept innervation; stabilisation (increase in half-life) of receptors in the clusters and decrease in the open time of the transmitter-activated ion channels; elimination of transmitter receptors from extrajunctional membranes; and development of synaptic folds.

In rats and chicks cholinesterase activity begins to develop at sites of nerve contact only when the muscle is activated (Lømo & Slater, 1980*b*) but in amphibia activity may not be required (Weldon, Moody Corbett & Cohen, 1981). Cholinesterase at the neuromuscular junction is made up of a mixture of different polymeric forms of the basic monomeric globular protein G1 (Massoulie & Bon, 1982). The largest molecule is the endplate-specific form A12, which has three blocks of four globular units held together by a collagen tail anchoring it to the basal lamina in the synaptic cleft. Muscles made up of different proportions of fast and slow twitch muscle fibres have characteristically different proportions of the different polymers and these differences can be reproduced by stimulating dener-vated rat muscles with different patterns of stimulation; a pattern mimic-king the discharge pattern found in motor neurons innervating fast muscle fibres reproduces the cholinesterase profile of a fast muscle and a slow stimulation regime reproduces the profile of a slow muscle (Lømo, Massou-lie & Vigny, 1985). These experiments show that cholinesterase is made and secreted by the muscle fibres and that its production and composition is controlled by the pattern of muscle fibre activity. With monoclonal antibodies it has been possible to show that several antigens other than cholinesterase are unique to the basal lamina at the adult neuromuscular junction (Chiu & Sanes, 1984; three examples have been given already viz. agrin, s-laminin and N-CAM) but the timing of their appearance does not coincide exactly with that of cholinesterase.

The decrease in the open time of channels at the junction is due to synthesis of synapse-specific acetylcholine receptors, which differ from the extrajunctional receptors in having one different subunit in each five-membered subunit ring, the γ unit being replaced by an ϵ unit (fig. 7.2; Mishima *et al.*, 1986; Schuetze & Role, 1987). Electrical activity in the muscle suppresses the synthesis of mRNA for extra-junctional acetylcho-line receptors by nuclei throughout the muscle fibre, but nuclei immediately beneath the nerve terminal continue to synthesise mRNA for junctional receptors (fig. 7.2; Merlie & Sanes, 1985). This points to a local chemical influence of the nerve on regulation of junctional receptor synthesis. A candidate for the substance is calcitonin-gene-related peptide, which is present in at least some motor neurons during development and can increase synthesis of AChRs in myotubes in culture (New & Mudge, 1986).

Embryonic and neonatal motor neurons make a variety of peptides which they do not express in adulthood and it is natural to wonder if they might play a part in the early interactions between motor neurons and muscle fibres. β-Endorphin is one such peptide (Haynes, Smyth & Zakar-ian, 1982). It appears to inhibit cholinesterase (Haynes & Smith, 1982) and its secretion by motor nerve terminals might help to increase the safety factor for transmission at developing junctions.

Electrical activity in the muscle plays an important role in synaptogene-sis: in addition to suppressing extrajunctional acetylcholine receptor syn-thesis, it makes the muscle fibre refractory to further innervation (Jansen *et al.*, 1973), stimulates the formation of folds in the postsynaptic membrane (Brenner, Meier & Widmer, 1983) and stimulates the accumulation of cholinesterase in the junctional cleft (Lømo & Slater, 1980*b*). For this reason, it seems likely that some of the properties of the developing muscle fibre, including long channel open times, low levels of cholinesterase, and high input resistance (due in part to the small fibre size) are designed specifically to increase the efficacy of synaptic transmission in the initial stages of synaptic development. The mechanisms by which activity effects the changes in the developing muscle cell are still unknown.

Synaptogenesis in the CNS

Much less is known about events in the development of synapses elsewhere in the nervous system, where single synapses are very much harder to isolate and manipulate. The process may differ from that at the neuromuscular junction in important respects. For example, postsynaptic structures can develop in the absence of their presynaptic axons both in ganglia (Smolen, 1981) and in the cerebellum (Rakic, 1975). Nearly all neurons receive many more than one synaptic input from a variety of different sources, each with its own transmitter. Any form of electrical signalling from inhibitory synapses, with a tendency to hyperpolarise the cell membrane, must be different from that in muscle. Furthermore, unlike the syncytial muscle fibre, neurons only have one nucleus to direct the manufacture of several transmitter receptor molecules. It is interesting that ribosomal RNA has been found in the dendrites of hippocampal neurons but not in their axons (see Chapter 5), and this may enable local synthesis of transmitter receptors in response to local signals (Gordon-Weeks, 1988).

Sensory receptor formation

The peripheral terminals of most sensory axons are closely associated with specialised receptor cells that take part in transducing a sensory stimulus into electrical impulses. The relationship between the sensory nerve and its end-organ has been studied in muscle spindles, Merkel cells and taste buds.

Muscle spindles cannot be detected in the adult rat if the afferents are removed at birth (Zelena, 1964). It is also known that muscle spindle primary afferents reach the developing muscle spindle before any of its motor axons (Milburn, 1973), so it is possible that myotubes contacted by the afferents are induced to develop into the specialised muscle fibres of the spindle, while myotubes contacted by motor axons develop into normal extrafusal muscle fibres. If the entry of afferents into developing muscle is delayed rather than prevented, hybrid muscle fibres develop in which the centre of the fibre in contact with the afferent has the typical appearance of an intrafusal fibre but the poles are large and look like normal extrafusal fibres (Werner, 1973).

In the case of innervation of Merkel cells (specialised touch receptors in the skin) it is known that the receptor cells pre-exist before arrival of the nerve and can develop partially in the nerve's absence (Scott, Cooper & Diamond, 1981). The Merkel cell afferent seeks out its target either by chemotropism or by random searching and recognition (English, Burgess & Norman, 1980).

Taste buds do not develop in the tongue at all if the IXth nerve on both sides is cut at birth (Hosley, Hughes & Oakley, 1987). The special sensory afferents in the nerve are therefore thought to induce formation of taste bud stem cells from the lingual epithelium, but it is not clear if the taste buds are induced from special progenitor cells. Reinnervation of denervated adult tongue by non-gustatory afferents of the vagus restores normal taste bud morphology (Zalewski, 1981), so the induction signal is not specific to the normal gustatory sensory axons.

The conclusion from these experiments is that the presence of sensory nerves is essential for the normal development of the sensory end-organs (and also for their maintenance in the adult). However, the nature of the signal from the sensory nerves is still unknown.

Neuron–glial relationships

As peripheral nerves develop and mature the larger axons become myelinated by their glial cells while the smaller axons remain unmyelinated. If myelinated nerves are cross-sutured with the distal segment of an unmyelinated nerve, the regenerating axons will become myelinated, whereas an unmyelinated nerve regenerating into a previously myelinated nerve remains unmyelinated (Simpson & Young, 1945). This means that the axons, rather than the glial cells, control the myelination. The signal for myelination may be in part causally related to axon diameter, since there is a good correlation between degree of myelination and diameter (Friede, 1972). A vivid demonstration of this is the development of myelination by the normally unmyelinated axons of postganglionic sympathetic neurons when, following partial denervation of their target tissues soon after birth, the remaining neurons and their axons increase in size (Voyvodic, 1989*b*).

Schwann cells secrete a basal lamina that encloses the entire Schwann cell–axon complex. This acellular stocking is needed if the Schwann cells are to myelinate their axons successfully (Sanes, 1989*b*) and it provides a persistent scaffolding after nerve degeneration to confine dividing Schwann cells and guide regrowing axons (see Chapter 12). Before myelination all Schwann cells express N-CAM, but after myelination N-CAM synthesis is down-regulated leaving only the unmyelinating Schwann cells (Remak cells) with N-CAM on their surface membranes (Jessen, Mirsky & Morgan, 1987).

Schwann cells in their turn influence the differentiation of axons during development. The excitable membrane of the axon is restricted to the nodal region of myelinated nerves by the Schwann cells, because saltatory conduction does not develop in axons if glial cells are absent, and saltatory conduction is replaced by continuous conduction if mature axons are demyelinated with diptheria toxin (Bostock & Sears, 1978).

Another cell type in peripheral nerves is the perineurial cell. These form an impermeable layer around the outside of each major nerve and nerve bundle that, together with the impermeable nature of the capillaries, provides the axons with a protected environment. These special cells arise from fibroblasts as a result of an interaction that needs the presence of both axons and Schwann cells (Sanes, 1989b; Bunge et al., 1989).

Many genetic abnormalities of peripheral and central myelination have been identified. In some of them the myelinating cell is at fault and in others the axon (Bray, Rasminsky & Aguayo, 1981).

Part 4

Modification of connections

Chapter 8

Nerve cell death

Introduction

Most of the different types of neuron in the vertebrate nervous system are subject to a period of cell death, which occurs shortly after axons begin to reach and activate their targets (Hamburger & Oppenheim, 1982). The extent of cell death for a given type of neuron is determined from estimates of the absolute number of neurons at a given site at different developmental stages. The number of neurons is found first to rise to a maximum as neurons proliferate and settle at their final destination, then to decline with the onset of cell death, and finally to reach a plateau when the period of death has passed. Death of the neurons is confirmed by the presence of degenerating nerve cell bodies during the decline in numbers of normal cells.

The proportion of cells that dies varies in the different parts of the nervous system. Death eliminates only a small fraction of the neurons at some sites but extensive death eliminating at least half of the total number of neurons generated can occur. Cell death is thus a major event in neuronal development, and there has been a succession of hypotheses about the purpose it might serve and its mechanism. The evidence discussed below points to cell death acting to leave behind only those neurons with quantitatively enough and qualitatively suitable pre- and post-synaptic connections. This seemingly wasteful process appears to have evolved in preference to accurate generation of neuron numbers and perfect guidance and targeting of outgrowing axons (Clarke, 1981). In nervous systems with very large numbers of cells such initial precision might be impossible. A mechanism involving competition and elimination of the least appropriate cells can achieve the same ends and, being more flexible, might provide a more suitable basis for rapid evolutionary changes in brain anatomy and function.

Specific proteins derived from target tissues are necessary for the survival of different kinds of embryonic neuron in tissue culture, and there is now convincing evidence that such 'trophic' factors are required for the survival of at least some neurons during development. Activity in the nerve–target pathways is another important part of the mechanism underlying cell death, and this may modulate the production and uptake of the trophic factors. Neurons may also require adequate afferent input for survival, either to enable the cells to be electrically active or to provide a further source of trophic factors.

Although their nervous systems contain far fewer cells than those of vertebrates, neuronal death also occurs in invertebrates. However, the extent of death is less and the purpose and mechanism may be different (Truman, 1984). Some neurons appear to be by-products of the generation of other neurons from precursor cells, or they may have a temporary role to play. A 'programmed' death then occurs that may not depend on lack of trophic factors or activity.

The purpose of cell death

Observations on the death of various classes of neuron during development in normal and experimental animals have led to suggestions of several different 'purposes' or reasons for cell death, including elimination of neurons whose axons fail to reach a target, scaling down of neuron numbers to match the size of a target or the size of a presynaptic pool, and the elimination of connection errors. More than one of these purposes may be in operation in specific cases of neuronal death. In addition, a temporary excess of neurons might have a positive role to play in some circumstances. For example muscle fibre numbers are regulated by the number of innervating motor neurons, fewer secondary myotubes being made for fewer innervating motor neurons (Ross, Duxson & Harris, 1987). The excess of motor neurons during development may therefore be needed to ensure the production of enough muscle fibres. Again some populations of neurons may disappear altogether having perhaps also served a temporary function (Chun, Nakamura & Shatz, 1987).

Elimination of neurons whose axons fail to reach a target

Nerve cell death was first observed in sensory ganglia and in motor neurons in the ventral horn of the spinal cord of chick embryos following removal of limb buds before they became innervated. This produced a virtually complete degeneration of all the neurons (motor neurons and dorsal root ganglion cells) that had been deprived of their targets in the limb (see Hamburger, 1980, for a review). When cell death in normal embryos was discovered subsequently in ganglia and the spinal cord (Hamburger & Levi-Montalcini, 1949), it was found to occur at the same time as the induced cell death and differed only in being less extensive. This suggested that the neurons that die are simply those that fail to reach a suitable target. This attractively simple idea may well account for neuronal death at some sites in the nervous system. For example, the sympathetic preganglionic motor neurons are generated as a uniform column of cells (the columns of Terni) on each side of the spinal cord, but at the cervical level these neurons appear to lack a target and subsequently degenerate. If the cervical cord is transplanted to the thoracic level some of the cells succeed in innervating ganglia and survive (Shieh, 1951). However, it has also been found that horseradish peroxidase injected into target tissues of somatic motor neurons and parasympathetic neurons just before cell death occurs can be detected subsequently in cells that die (Lamb, 1976; Landmesser & Pilar, 1976). This means that failure to reach a suitable target cannot be the only reason for cell death.

Scaling down neuron numbers to match the size of the target

Neuronal death in the sensory ganglia and cord at segmental levels that innervate the limbs is less extensive than at the levels that innervate the trunk regions, where there is much less tissue to be innervated. Moreover if extra limbs are grafted onto early embryos in limb-innervating regions there is less neuronal death than normal (Hollyday & Hamburger, 1976). Conversely, nearly all motor neurons are lost from the lateral motor column of the mutant chick 'limbless' (Lanser & Fallon, 1984). These observations are consistent with the hypothesis that a given target tissue in some way supports the survival of only a limited number of the neurons that initially innervate it. Thus, cell death could be a means of matching appropriately the sizes of independently generated pre- and post-synaptic cell populations by limiting survival of the pre-synaptic cells (Cowan, 1973; fig. 8.1). Strong support for this hypothesis has come from an experiment in which chick lumbosacral cords were transplanted into quails and quail lumbosacral cords into chicks before the limbs became innervated (Tanaka & Landmesser, 1986*b*). Chicks are larger than quails and have more muscle fibres. It was found that more quail motor neurons survived in the chick than in the quail, and fewer chick motor neurons survived in the quail than in the chick. Overall there was a strong correlation between the number of motor neurons surviving and the number of muscle fibres.

Quantitative loss of neurons to match the number of target sites also occurs in the dorsal root ganglion cell population. If one limb bud is removed from *Xenopus* tadpoles, the single developing limb can become innervated by the motor and sensory axons of both sides. The total number

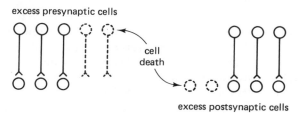

Fig. 8.1. Possible matching of pre- and post-synaptic cell populations by cell death (1:1 matching shown here for simplicity).

of sensory ganglion cells surviving is the same as the normal number for one side (Lamb, Ferns & Klose., 1989). It seems that one limb can only support a limited number of ganglion cells. However, quite a different result was obtained for motor neurons (see below).

Scaling down neuron numbers to match the size of the presynaptic neuron pool

A test of whether motor neuron death is influenced by the amount of presynaptic input was carried out by Oppenheim and his coworkers, who eliminated sensory inputs by excising the neural crest and also removed other descending inputs by transecting the spinal cord (Okada & Oppenheim, 1984). When both these inputs were eliminated there was a considerable increase in the amount of motor neuron cell death, implying that presynaptic inputs do influence survival of motor neurons. A similar result was obtained for motor neurons in the frog (Davis, Constantine-Paton & Schorr, 1983), and a similar partial dependency on presynaptic input for survival of parasympathetic neurons has been seen in the ciliary ganglion of the chick (Furber, Oppenheim & Prevette, 1987).

Observations on neuronal death in neonatal rats following injury to the optic nerve suggest that postsynaptic and presynaptic population matching may regulate the survival of retinal ganglion cells (fig. 8.2). Severing the optic nerve before the chiasm reduces death in the other eye in those ganglion cells that project ipsilaterally from the temporal retina, presumably because removal of the axon terminals of one eye leaves relatively more target for the remaining axons (Jeffery & Perry, 1982). Section of the optic tract on the central side of the chiasm also leads to less death in the same ganglion cells, in this case possibly because these ganglion cells receive more presynaptic input from the other neurons in the retina following the degeneration of the injured neurons (Linden & Perry, 1982).

Elimination of connection errors

An experiment by Lamb (1980, 1981) cast doubt on the idea that death reduces motor neuron pool sizes to match the size of their targets. Lamb succeeded in diverting the outgrowing nerves from one side of the spinal cord into the developing contralateral leg in *Xenopus* tadpoles. The surprising result was a normal-sized leg musculature innervated by twice as many motor neurons, implying there was no increase in the amount of cell death on either side of the cord. This result is at variance with the chick–quail chimaera experiments that demonstrated a strong inverse relationship between motor neuron death and target size (see above), and it calls for some other reason for motor neuron death, at least in frogs.

A plausible alternative purpose for cell death, which might explain Lamb's observations, is that it is a means of eliminating qualitative as well as quantitative errors in pre- and post-synaptic connections. The additional

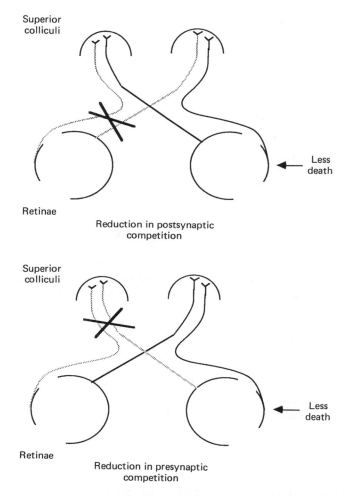

Fig. 8.2. Reduced cell death in temporal retina following neonatal
transection of either optic nerve (above) or optic tract (below).

evidence that this might be so consists of several clear instances where
labelling neurons with tracers has revealed connections in the developing
animal that are not present in the adult and that are removed by the death of
the neurons making them (fig. 8.3).

First, in the chick embryo, HRP injected into the eye revealed that axons
projecting to the retina arise initially not only from the appropriate
contralateral isthmo-optic nucleus, but also from a small number of cells in
the ipsilateral nucleus (fig. 8.3a). Most of the ectopic neurons, and all of the
ipsilateral neurons, are removed by cell death (Clarke & Cowan, 1976).

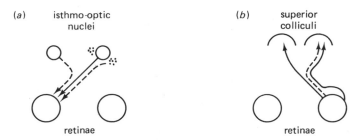

Fig. 8.3. Connection errors (shown as dotted lines) which are removed by cell death. (*a*) Ectopic and ipsilateral connections from isthmo-optic nuclei to retina in chick embryos. (*b*) Ipsilateral projections from nasal retina in neonatal rats.

Secondly, in neonatal rats there are erroneous projections from nasal retina to the ipsilateral superior colliculus. Using a technique of double labelling, Jeffery & Perry (1982) were able to show that these projections are removed by cell death (fig. 8.3*b*). Thirdly, topographic targeting errors in the contralateral projection from the eye to the colliculus are removed during the period of retinal ganglion cell death (O'Leary, Fawcett & Cowan, 1986). Fourthly, the segregation of retinal ganglion cell afferents into their characteristic layers in the lateral geniculate body begins in the Rhesus monkey at the time of retinal ganglion cell death (Rakic, 1986), and the somatotopic projection of motor neurons to the gluteus muscle of the toad develops during the period of motor neuron death (Bennett & Lavidis, 1982). These findings suggest that incorrectly projecting neurons are being eliminated to create the ordered adult pattern of connections.

Mechanism of nerve cell death

Target-derived trophic factors
Most of the observations of cell death in the vertebrate nervous system are consistent with the hypothesis that target tissues release specific 'trophic' factors that are necessary for the survival of their neurons. It is believed that neurons that do not take up a sufficient quantity of the trophic factors during development are the neurons that die. The failure of neurons to obtain adequate amounts of target-released growth factors provides an obvious explanation for the death of neurons that are in relative excess compared with their target cells, since there would be competition between the neurons for a limited amount of factor available from the target. It can also explain the death of neurons contacting the wrong targets, if either the axons cannot make or maintain adequate contacts with the incorrect target in order to gain access to the factor, or if the factor is unsuitable for the errant neurons.

Definitive evidence for a role for trophic factors in cell death requires isolation and characterisation of such factors and experimental verification of their importance. This was first achieved satisfactorily for Nerve Growth Factor. NGF is a protein that was first isolated from a mouse sarcoma following observation of its growth-stimulatory effects on sympathetic ganglia in chick embryos (see Levi-Montalcini & Calissano, 1979). In the course of isolation attempts, snake venom was used as a source of enzymes to find out if the active agent was a protein or nucleic acid. The venom itself turned out to have the same action as the tumour and subsequently a range of tissues (e.g. male mouse submaxillary salivary glands, guinea pig prostate gland; reviewed by Thoenen & Barde, 1980) were shown to be similarly active. The reason for the extraordinarily high concentration of NGF in these tissues is not clear but its presence did facilitate the isolation of the molecule. Only recently have techniques become sensitive enough to detect NGF in the target tissues of sensory and sympathetic neurons (Ebendal *et al.*, 1980). A further step in that direction is the capability of detecting mRNA for NGF in very small samples of tissue (Heumann *et al.*, 1984; Heumann, 1987).

The evidence that NGF is obligatory for the survival of sympathetic and sensory neurons in the animal is very strong. NGF injected into neonatal rats prevents both normal and also experimentally-induced death in the sympathetic ganglia, and in embryonic chicks it prevents cell death in the dorsal root ganglia (Hamburger, Brunso Bechtold & Yip, 1981). Moreover, uptake and transport mechanisms specific for NGF exist in sympathetic and sensory axons (see Thoenen & Barde, 1980). However, the most convincing evidence for a role for NGF in the normal animal is the phenomenon of immunosympathectomy: the death of all sympathetic ganglion cells when NGF antiserum is injected into neonatal rats (Levi-Montalcini & Cohen, 1960). Sensory neurons are also killed by exposure to NGF antibodies in the embryo (Johnson *et al.*, 1980). Recent work suggests that it may also be needed by some neurons in the CNS (see Marx, 1986). The evidence for a continuing role for NGF in the adult is given in Chapter 11.

The mechanism of action of NGF is not yet clear. Injection of NGF into the cytoplasm or nucleus of NGF-dependent cells does not produce the same effects as outside application, nor do intracellularly-injected antibodies disrupt its action. It appears that the molecule has to be taken up by NGF-specific receptors, whose structure is known (Radeke *et al.*, 1987), and delivered to the cell body by retrograde axoplasmic transport. At some stage some form of second messenger must be made. Recently it has been found that the product of a *ras* oncogene, ras p21 protein, can promote the survival of both NGF-dependent and NGF-independent neurons *in vitro*, if the protein is allowed to get into the cells by exposing them to it in the presence of trypsin (Borasio *et al.*, 1989). This oncogene protein is related to

GTP-binding proteins and it is thus possible that they are the common site of action of a variety of growth factors, both those known and those as yet uncharacterised. Somewhat surprisingly it seems that NGF may prevent cells making 'suicide' molecules in addition to just helping them to manufacture useful ones, for the rapid death of NGF-dependent neurons when NGF is withdrawn can be prevented by applying agents that block protein synthesis (see Barnes, 1988).

Another trophic molecule similar to NGF is Brain-Derived Neurotrophic Factor (BDNF), which has been purified from brain on the basis of its ability to support survival of embryonic sensory neurons *in vitro* (Barde, 1988; 1989). It appears to be a factor involved in the survival of some sensory neurons *in vivo*, for injections of BDNF into quail embryos in extremely small amounts increase the survival of neurons in dorsal root and nodose ganglia (Hofer & Barde, 1988).

Direct evidence for a role for factors other than NGF and BDNF in promoting survival of other neurons *in vivo* is lacking. Nevertheless it seems very likely that neurons throughout the nervous system are dependent for their survival on specific growth factors, and that the target cells of the neurons are a source of these (Purves, 1988). Thus extracts of embryonic muscle or supernatants of muscle cultures enhance survival of motor neurons in culture (Bennett, Lai & Nurcombe, 1980; Dohrmann *et al.*, 1986, 1987; Smith *et al.*, 1986; reviewed by Henderson, 1988) and *in vivo* (Oppenheim *et al.*, 1988); extracts of the ciliary body enhance the survival of the parasympathetic ciliary ganglion (Nishi & Berg, 1981); and medium conditioned by cultures of tectum promotes the survival of retinal ganglion cells (Nurcombe & Bennett, 1981). One difficulty in isolating the factors is the very low concentrations that may exist in the tissues (Barde, 1988). NGF itself might still be uncharacterised but for the lucky and unexplained high concentrations found in some tissues, for it otherwise exists in very small amounts indeed. Further difficulties in the assay systems include the presence of non-specific factors such as laminin, which can provide a degree of trophic support (Dohrmann *et al.*, 1986), or nonspecific toxic agents which can obscure any survival or axon growth-supporting action in the extracts.

There are two other well-characterised molecules that can promote nerve cell survival *in vitro*: Fibroblast Growth Factor (FGF) and Ciliary Neurotrophic Factor (CNTF). FGF is a mitogen for fibroblasts, myoblasts and endothelial cells; it can act as a mesoderm-inducing agent in amphibian blastulae, but it also promotes survival of ciliary ganglion neurons *in vivo* if an exogenous store is implanted in the chick chorio-allantoic membrane (Dreyer *et al.*, 1989). CNTF *in vitro* supports survival of most peripheral neurons (Barbin, Manthorpe & Varon, 1984) and initiates the development of type 2 astrocytes in the rat optic nerve (Lillien *et al.*, 1988; see Chapter 3). FGF and CNTF differ from NGF and BDNF in that they are present in relatively high concentrations *in vivo* and so would not seem at first sight to be an object of competition at the time of naturally occurring cell death (Barde, 1988). Perhaps the limiting factor is not the amount of trophic material but the ability of neurons to gain access to it (Oppenheim, 1989).

Role of electrical activity

The death of motor neurons and sympathetic neurons appears to be modulated by electrical activity of their target tissues. Direct stimulation of the muscle causes more motor neuron death than normal (Oppenheim & Nunez, 1982), while inactivation by the postsynaptic blocking agents curare or α-bungarotoxin or by the presynaptic blocking agent botulinum toxin is an effective means of preventing motor neuron death (Pittman & Oppenheim, 1978; Laing & Prestige, 1978). Similar observations have been made on the innervation of sympathetic ganglia, where it has been found that blockade of transmission also causes less death in the preganglionic motor nuclei (Oppenheim, Maderdrut & Wells, 1982). These results are consistent with the idea that inactive target cells produce sufficient growth factor to support all neurons in contact with the target, but that with the onset of innervation and activation less factor is produced and some neurons subsequently die.

Lack of target-released factors may also be involved in the death of neurons with incorrect or insufficient presynaptic inputs if presynaptically misconnected neurons are electrically less active and the uptake or utilisation of target-released factors is modulated by electrical activity. However, it is also possible that presynaptic inputs provide their own trophic factors to the neurons (see below), or that neurons have a direct metabolic requirement for electrical activity during this phase of development.

Other trophic factors

A dependence on trophic support from presynaptic sources is suggested by the observation that extracts of target (muscle) and BDNF, which is of CNS origin, can act synergistically to enhance the survival of proprioceptive sensory neurons in culture (Davies, Thoenen & Barde, 1986). Lack of trophic factors from glia or some other source may explain the cell death in the lateral geniculate nucleus that occurs before any afferent input has arrived or any efferent connections have been made (Williams & Rakic, 1988), but programmed cell death could be operating here. Sex hormones have been shown to affect the survival of motor neurons innervating the bulbocavernosus muscle in rats (Breedlove & Arnold, 1983a,b), which raises the possibility that other classes of neuron might require certain hormones for survival.

The various possible factors that may be involved during the process of nerve cell death are summarised in fig. 8.4.

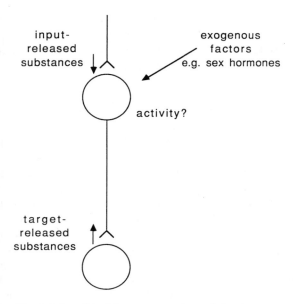

Fig. 8.4. Possible factors preventing cell death.

Neuronal death in invertebrates

Investigation of neuronal death in several invertebrate species has revealed that the nerve's target tissue does not play the same key role that it does in vertebrates. In grasshopper embryos a stereotyped pattern of cell division in the segmental ganglia generates thoracic motor neurons which innervate the legs, and homologous neurons in the abdomen which have no tissue to innervate and which die. However, removal of the limb buds does *not* cause the death of those neurons in the thoracic ganglia that would normally innervate leg muscles (Goodman & Bate, 1981). This means that the absence of target tissue is probably not the cause of death of neurons in the abdominal ganglion, but whether there is some other environmental cue or whether the cells are intrinsically specified to die is not known. A similar kind of neuronal death occurs in the nematode, where again there are stereotyped patterns of cell division followed by death of specific, apparently superfluous, neurons. The possibility of intrinsically programmed death is suggested by the observation that the neurons die even before they establish processes, but again a local environmental cue cannot be ruled out as yet (Sulston & Horvitz, 1977).

A factor that may be important in the control of neuronal death in some invertebrates is presynaptic input. In the locust visual system a small proportion of neurons in the optic lobe die during normal development. If the retina is prevented from projecting to the optic lobe there is an increased degeneration of optic lobe neurons, whereas an experimentally increased projection produces less cell death (Anderson, Edwards & Palka, 1980; Truman, 1984). Thus it is likely that some cells in the optic lobe die during normal development because they are not utilised by retinal afferents.

During metamorphosis from pupa to adult various neurons and muscles may die. In the moth *Manduca* death of some motor neurons is controlled by the level of steroid moulting hormone. As the levels of the hormone fall following the moult the motor neurons, which appear to have now become dependent on it, die but can be rescued by injections of appropriate steroid (Truman, 1984).

Chapter 9

Excess connections and their elimination

Introduction

Cajal and his associates were the first to present evidence that there might be an initial excess of connections in the developing nervous system. In CNS tissue stained by the Golgi method it was apparent that many more spines were present on the dendrites of some neurons during development than in the adult. It was also noticed that muscle fibres in neonatal animals appeared to be contacted by branches of several axons, in contrast to adult fibres which were innervated invariably by a single axon. Further research on this phenomenon awaited its rediscovery more than 50 years later, when electrophysiological investigations of neonatal muscles revealed that individual muscle fibres were innervated initially by more than one axon (fig. 9.1). It has since been shown that elimination of the excess inputs requires activity in the muscle and may involve competition between the separate inputs for a muscle-associated growth stimulus.

A similar excess of presynaptic inputs in neonatal animals has also been demonstrated physiologically on neurons of autonomic ganglia and on Purkinje cells of the cerebellum. Direct visualisation of these excess inputs has so far not been possible, but at many other places in the CNS axon branching can be seen to be initially more diffuse than in the mature nervous system. The most well-known examples are from loci in the visual system, in particular the lateral geniculate nucleus, the superior colliculus and layer IV of the visual cortex, where the axon terminals corresponding to each eye are in discrete bands in the adult but are intermingled in embryonic or neonatal animals. Excess or aberrant axon branches have been observed at several other sites in the developing CNS, including the corpus callosum and the pyramidal tract.

Another example of synapse reorganisation concerns the connections that relay visual information from layer IV to the other layers in the visual cortex. Diffuse branching of the axons that project from layer IV has not been visualised directly, but its presence can be inferred from the receptive fields of the neurons, that is from the visual stimuli that make the neurons respond. Initially the neurons respond to a wider range of visual stimuli than they do in the adult, but a fine tuning to specific stimuli gradually

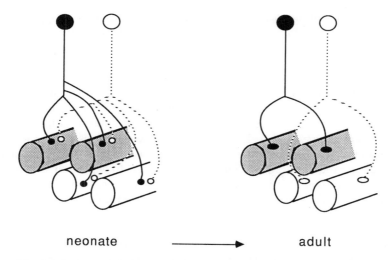

neonate ⟶ adult

Fig. 9.1. Polyneuronal innervation of muscle fibres by motor neurons at birth and its elimination to leave each muscle fibre with only a single innervating axon in the adult.

develops and can be modified by visual experience only during a certain 'critical' period. This fine tuning may be achieved by functional suppression of some inputs, as well as by axon withdrawal. Other examples of critical periods that may have excess connections as their basis are considered at the end of this chapter.

It is important to note that in all these cases the phase of cell death for the presynaptic neurons is over before the excess presynaptic inputs are eliminated. It follows that the excess inputs are a consequence of diffuse branching of the presynaptic axons rather than a consequence of an excess of presynaptic neurons. The extra branches develop presumably in response to local growth stimuli at the time when connections are first established and they are eliminated when they fail to make stable synaptic contacts.

Multiple innervation at the neuromuscular junction

The presence of more than one functional input at the neuromuscular junction of neonatal rat muscle fibres was first detected by Redfern, who was recording *in vitro* from muscle fibres in which the endplate potentials had been reduced to subthreshold levels with curare. Under such conditions the endplate potential of an adult muscle fibre has a relatively constant amplitude independent of the stimulus size, but in the neonatal muscle endplate potentials of individual fibres show several consistent stepwise increments as more axons are stimulated in the muscle nerve (Redfern, 1970). The presence of excess axonal branches was confirmed by demonstrations that individual motor units were several times larger than in the adult (Bagust, Lewis & Westerman, 1973; Brown, Jansen & Van Essen, 1976), and by visualisation of intramuscular nerves and nerve terminals in the light and electron microscopes (Brown *et al.*, 1976; Riley, 1976; Korneliussen & Jansen, 1976).

Interest has now centred on explaining how all axonal branches except one are eliminated from the neuromuscular junction in most muscles in vertebrates. As with neuronal death, the precise nature of the mechanism has not been established, but a number of conclusions about the elimination process have been made: elimination occurs by retraction rather than degeneration of branches; elimination appears to depend on a competition between axons for muscle fibres; and the competition is modulated by postsynaptic activity and by type- and place-specific 'matching' of motor neurons and muscle fibres.

Most eliminated branches are retracted

It was originally thought that the excess branches at the neuromuscular junction were removed by degeneration (Rosenthal & Taraskevich, 1977), and this may be the fate of some relatively long excess branches that occur outside the endplate region (Jenq, Chung & Coggeshall, 1986). However, it seems that any nerve degeneration seen in neonatal muscles is insufficient to account for the removal of the excess branches (Bixby, 1981). Swollen nerve terminals that are not in contact with an endplate can be seen in the light microscope during the elimination period (Riley, 1977), and in the electron microscope it appears that axonal structural components are being resorbed at such 'retraction bulbs' (Riley, 1981).

Competition for muscle fibres

The fact that in mammalian muscles elimination of excess axonal inputs proceeds until exactly one axon remains in contact with each muscle fibre has given rise to the idea of a competitive interaction between the nerve terminals for occupancy of muscle fibres. If, instead of competing for muscle fibres, neurons simply lost at random a proportion of their terminals, some muscle fibres would be completely denervated and others would become permanently innervated by several axons. Neither of these possibilities occurs in normal mammalian muscles (Brown *et al.*, 1976).

Further evidence for a competitive interaction between the nerve terminals was provided by experiments in which neonatal muscles were partly denervated and then allowed to mature. In the rat soleus (Brown *et al.*, 1976) and lumbrical muscles (Betz, Caldwell & Ribchester, 1980) this resulted in motor units in the adult that were larger than normal; thus the normal loss of excess branches had been attenuated, presumably because removal of some motor axons had reduced the competition for muscle fibres.

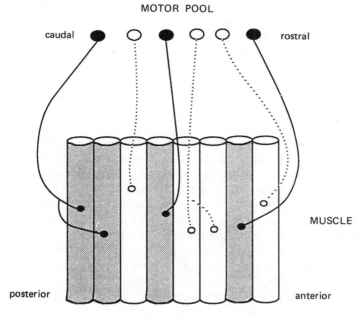

Fig. 9.2. Distribution of motor axons in muscle illustrating type-specificity and place-specificity.

The outcome of a competition between individual terminals may depend on how many extra branches their parent neurons are trying to support. Experiments on reinnervated adult muscles showed that the safety factor for transmission was lower in motor units that were larger than normal and higher in smaller units (Slack & Hopkins, 1982; Pockett & Slack, 1983). Furthermore, foreign motor axons growing into a normally innervated muscle can evict a normal terminal from its endplate, presumably because the normal terminals are at a competitive disadvantage compared with the foreign nerves, which initially have few terminal branches to support (Bixby & Van Essen, 1979). The nerve terminals of synapses that have developed from sprouts in a partially denervated muscle appear to be at a similar disadvantage when the original axons regenerate to their endplates (Brown & Ironton, 1978).

Type-matching and place-matching
Muscles are made up of different types of muscle fibre, but in the adult all the fibres of a motor unit are of the same type (Edstrom & Kugelberg, 1968). Motor neurons innervating similar types of fibre have similar properties (Burke, 1981), which indicates that there is a 'type-matching' of some motor neurons and muscle fibres (fig. 9.2). Similarly there is a 'place-

matching' (somatotopic projection) of neurons to fibres in some muscles, with the rostro-caudal axis of the motor neuron pool mapping to some extent with the posterior–anterior axis of the muscle (Brown & Booth, 1983; fig. 9.2). What role does the elimination of excess branches play in establishing type- and place-matching?

In the soleus muscles of the rat and rabbit the fibres of each motor unit are already homogeneous before synapse elimination is completed (Thompson, Sutton & Riley, 1984; Gordon & Van Essen, 1985), but in the IVth lumbrical muscle of the rat the muscle fibres of the motor units are more heterogeneous before the period of elimination and become less so during elimination (Jones, Ridge & Rowlerson, 1987a). Moreover, there is no evidence that the fibres of the motor units undergo conversion of their type at this time (Jones, Ridge & Rowlerson, 1987b), so it is possible that in this muscle the homogeneity of fibre type within a motor unit is established by selective elimination of terminals that are incorrectly matched to fibres.

Examination of the somatotopic ordering of motor units before and after synapse elimination has been carried out in frogs (Bennett & Lavidis, 1986) and in mammals (Bennett & Lavidis, 1984; Brown & Booth, 1983; Laskowski & High, 1989). In both cases some degree of place-specificity exists before elimination; however, the precision of the somatotopic projection is improved by the elimination process, indicating that better positionally-matched terminals are more likely to survive.

The role of activity

Several experiments have demonstrated the importance of electrical activity in the elimination of multiple innervation at the neuromuscular junction. The rate of elimination is accelerated by direct muscle stimulation (O'Brien, Ostberg & Vrbova, 1978). High frequency bursts of activity are more effective than a steady stimulation that delivers the same number of impulses (Thompson, 1983). Elimination is slowed or prevented when activity is reduced by various means (Benoit & Changeux, 1975; Thompson, Kuffler & Jansen, 1979; Brown, Holland & Hopkins, 1981; Duxson, 1982; Callaway & Van Essen, 1989).

There have been several suggestions for the mechanisms whereby postsynaptic activity regulates axon branch survival. It was once postulated that a muscle-released proteolytic enzyme might digest axon terminals and be released in smaller quantities when fibres are inactive (O'Brien, Ostberg & Vrbova, 1980). More recently it has been suggested that the protease is inside the nerve terminal and is activated by Ca^{2+} entry when the terminal is depolarised by action potentials (Vrbova, 1988). To explain the effect of postsynaptic activity it has been suggested that K^+ released by active muscle fibres further depolarises the nerve terminals and thereby increases Ca^{2+} entry and activity of the protease.

An alternative suggestion is that activity modulates the synthesis, release or degradation of a growth stimulus rather than a growth inhibitor. The substance could be a growth factor released from the junctional membrane, possibly identical to that for which the neurons are thought to compete for their survival earlier in development. Evidence for this possibility is the observation that locally applied NGF can promote survival of individual sympathetic nerve branches in tissue culture (Campenot, 1977). Alternatively the substance could be a component of the extracellular matrix of the endplate that influences nerve terminal growth by a contact-mediated interaction. This latter possibility is consistent with observations of elimination of multiple innervation in living reinnervated adult muscle: it was found that acetylcholine receptor density decreased beneath nerve terminals prior to their elimination, suggesting that lack of receptors or of molecules co-localised with them (or also of substances released near them) causes terminal withdrawal (Rich & Lichtman, 1989).

Experiments to determine the role of *presynaptic* activity in the elimination of multiple innervation at the neuromuscular junction have produced conflicting results. The terminals of stimulated motor axons have an advantage over unstimulated terminals both in neonatal rat muscles (Ridge & Betz, 1984) and in adult rat muscles that have multiply-innervated fibres following reinnervation (Ribchester & Taxt, 1983; Ribchester, 1988). In contrast, the terminals of axons made inactive by tetrodotoxin plugs have an advantage over active terminals in neonatal rabbit muscles (Callaway, Soha & Van Essen, 1987). In the CNS it appears that the more active inputs are retained in favour of less active ones, possibly because of a mechanism, based on the N-methyl-D-aspartate (NMDA) receptor, that stabilises the postsynaptic membrane of active synapses (see pp.104–5); these receptors do not exist at the vertebrate neuromuscular junction.

Adult multiply-innervated muscle fibres

A few mammalian muscles have a proportion of stable, multiply-innervated fibres and multiple innervation is common in adult avian muscles. Multiple innervation can also persist in fibres that have been reinnervated in different species. There have been various observations and experiments on these tissues aimed at elucidating the mechanism of the competitive interaction between motor nerves that occurs in the neonate.

A mammalian muscle that is multiply innervated in the adult is the rat *levator ani*. Multiple innervation is modulated in some unknown way by the level of circulating androgens: castration lowers the amount of polyinnervation, an effect that can be counteracted by androgen administration. The amount of polyinnervation remains high if the androgens are withdrawn once the animal is adult, so the dependence on sex hormones occurs during a limited time period (Jordan, Letinsky & Arnold, 1989*a,b*).

Competition leading to a reduction in synaptic effectiveness has been demonstrated between two foreign nerves implanted onto a denervated muscle in adult frogs. Transmission at individual synapses on fibres that are innervated by both nerves is less effective than on fibres that receive inputs from only one nerve (Grinnell, Letinsky & Rheuben, 1979). Such partial suppression has not been observed in mammalian twitch muscle fibres (Soha, Yo & Van Essen, 1987).

The spacing of synapses along the length of multiply-innervated fibres is an intriguing phenomenon. In adult rats a foreign nerve implanted on a denervated muscle produces multiply-innervated fibres with endplates spaced randomly along the individual fibres. Muscle activity is required to eliminate these endplates (Lømo & Slater, 1980a), and there appears to be a selective elimination of closely spaced inputs (Kuffler, Thompson & Jansen, 1980). A similar effect is seen for the elimination of postsynaptic specialisations if the foreign nerve is cut and the muscle is stimulated directly (Lømo, Pockett & Sommerschild, 1988). This apparent distance-dependent effect may reflect a limited capacity of the active muscle fibres to maintain postsynaptic specialisations along a given length of fibre. A similar conclusion was suggested by the observation that paralysis of chick embryos with curare produces regularly spaced synapses on muscle fibres that would normally be singly innervated and decreases the spacing between synapses on fibres that are normally multiply innervated (Gordon *et al.*, 1974). Direct stimulation of the nerves to developing embryonic chick hindlimb muscles can also alter the pattern of innervation: a 'slow' pattern of activity (continuous stimulation at 0.5 Hz) produces multiple synaptic sites on muscle fibres that would normally be singly innervated (Toutant *et al.*, 1980). Thus the pattern of activation appears to determine which muscle fibres develop and retain a distributed innervation.

A model for synapse elimination at the neuromuscular junction
Fig. 9.3 summarises the available observations on synapse elimination at the neuromuscular junction by illustrating schematically the gradual loss of attractiveness of the endplate brought about by postsynaptic activity and the withdrawal of axons that lose contact with the endplate. If it is assumed that increased contact with the endplate increases axon branch survival, positive feedback could stabilise a larger terminal and destabilise a smaller terminal, and this could lead to the elimination of some terminals (Purves & Lichtman, 1980). The effectiveness of the feedback would have to be very great to explain why one and only one terminal invariably survives at each endplate, so it is possible that other important variables controlling synaptic elimination at the neuromuscular junction have yet to be identified. It will be seen later in this chapter that correlated pre- and post-synaptic activity may play an important role in stabilising synapses in the CNS. While there is as yet no evidence for this at the neuromuscular junction an interaction of this nature may be necessary to prevent the last remaining nerve terminal from eliminating itself.

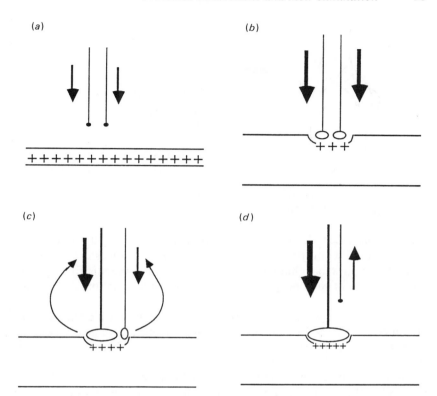

Fig. 9.3. One possible model for activity-modulated neuronal competition at the motor endplate. Amount and distribution of nerve terminal survival factor associated with a given muscle fibre is indicated by plus signs. Amount and direction of supply of materials from cell body is indicated by straight arrows. (*a*) Muscle fibre is initially very 'innervatable'. (*b*) Activity after functional contact (here by two axons) reduces 'innervatability' to a single site. (*c*) Activity may further reduce the availability of the growth/survival factor from the muscle. Curved arrows indicate that the terminal with the greater amount of contact with the postsynaptic site gains an enhanced supply and so grows by positive feedback. Conversely, the smaller terminal shrinks. (*d*) The terminal which loses all contact with the muscle is withdrawn.

Excess presynaptic inputs in autonomic ganglia

Graded stimulation of preganglionic axons and intracellular recording from ganglion cells revealed that the cells of the submandibular ganglion are innervated by up to five preganglionic fibres, but by 40 days of age the adult state of one axonal input per ganglion cell is established. When the synaptic boutons of the preganglionic axons were stained and counted in the light microscope, it was apparent that the total number of boutons on

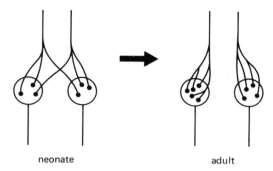

Fig. 9.4. Elimination of multiple innervation in the submandibular ganglion of the rat.

the cells increased throughout the period during which the number of inputs from different preganglionic axons on each cell was declining (fig. 9.4). This implies that elimination of some inputs allows redistribution and concentration of each preganglionic axon on fewer ganglion cells (Lichtman, 1977).

Neurons in the guinea pig superior cervical ganglion, which in the adult are innervated by 6–7 separate preganglionic axons, have nearly twice as many axonal inputs in the immature animal. The inputs in the neonate arise from an average of four contiguous spinal cord segmental levels, whereas in the adult they arise from less than three (Lichtman & Purves, 1980). Thus it is possible that graded segmental labels are involved in the competitive removal of excess inputs from ganglion cells. This view is strengthened by experiments (summarised by Njå and his colleagues – Leistol *et al.*, 1986) on the pattern of connections formed on reinnervation or partial denervation of ganglia of mature guinea pigs. There appeared to be graded affinities between terminals of preganglionic fibres and cells in the superior cervical ganglion. Also preganglionic axons with many connections appeared to be at a competitive disadvantage compared with those with fewer connections.

In the rabbit ciliary ganglion the postsynaptic cells are contacted initially by 4–5 axons, but in the adult this is reduced to a range of 1–5. There is a strong correlation between the number of inputs and the number of dendrites possessed by the adult but not by the neonatal ganglion cells, suggesting that the separate inputs are segregated onto separate dendrites during development. Thus competition for separate dendrites rather than for an entire neuron may allow multiple inputs to survive on adult nerve cells (Hume & Purves, 1981). Decreases in the amount of activity in the pathways to the ganglion slow the rate of removal of excess branches (Jackson, 1983).

It is apparent that elimination and rearrangement of branches in autonomic ganglia are controlled by factors similar to those at work at the neuromuscular junction: competition for synaptic sites modulated by the degree of activity, the degree of 'chemo-affinity' between various possible synaptic partners and the relative sizes of terminal tree supported by the competing neurons.

Excess connections in the CNS
Evidence for the extra connections in the brain during development takes several forms. In the cerebellum, extra inputs similar to those on muscle fibres can be demonstrated on Purkinje cells using physiological techniques. Diffuse extra branches can be visualised on the terminals of axons in the visual pathway and wholly aberrant branches that travel considerable distances can also be seen in several parts of the brain using histological techniques. At higher levels of the visual system and elsewhere in the brain the receptive field properties of neurons betray the existence of connections that may be lost as the animal matures. The changes that occur in most if not all of these connections during development are dependent upon the electrical activity in the pathways.

Multiple climbing fibre inputs on Purkinje cells
Purkinje cells in the adult rat cerebellum are innervated by one climbing fibre from the inferior olive but in the neonate 2–3 climbing fibre inputs can be detected by recording from Purkinje cells and applying graded stimulation to the inferior olive (Crepel, Mariani & Delhaye Bouchaud, 1976). These multiple climbing fibre inputs persist in various cerebellar mouse mutants and experimental animals that have in common a failure in the formation of parallel fibre synapses on the Purkinje dendrites. It has been suggested that the parallel fibre synapses may strengthen the competitive interaction among the climbing fibres by decreasing the supply of some trophic factor to the climbing fibres from the Purkinje cells (Crepel, 1982).

Excess axon branches in the visual pathway
Several histological methods based on axonal transport have been used to delineate the distribution of axon terminals in the visual pathways. A radioactively labelled amino acid can be injected into one eye, from where it is transported along the axons of the retinal ganglion cells to their terminals in the lateral geniculate nucleus (LGN) and superior colliculus; subsequent autoradiography of sections of the brain can then reveal the gross distribution of the terminals from one eye in the LGN and superior colliculus. Some label is also transferred to the cells in the LGN and thence to the terminals of these cells in layer IV of the visual cortex, where it can also be detected by so-called 'transneuronal' autoradiography. If one eye is injected in the adult the terminals in the LGN, superior colliculus and visual cortex are revealed as discrete bands of label interdigitated with equal-sized unlabelled bands corresponding to the uninjected eye. During development, however, the

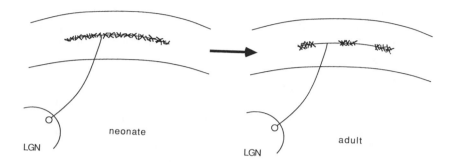

Fig. 9.5. Possible mode of development of ocular dominance columns in the cortex. Terminal branching of an afferent from the lateral geniculate nucleus to layer IV in the visual cortex of the neonate (left) becomes restricted to bands in the adult (right).

terminals are initially intermingled and gradually segregate into bands, by birth in the LGN and superior colliculus and by several weeks of age in the visual cortex (Rakic, 1977*a,b*). By recording from neurons in layer IV it is possible to demonstrate that there is a correlated functional segregation of the inputs from each eye into 'ocular dominance columns' (Hubel, Wiesel & Le Vay, 1977). Staining of terminal arborisations of individual geniculate afferents in the cortex of adults (by the injection of HRP into single fibres) has shown a pattern of branches in which areas of dense projection are separated by areas largely devoid of branches (Wiesel, 1982). In all likelihood the branch-free areas correspond to regions of the terminal arborisation that are lost during development of ocular dominance columns (fig. 9.5). Similarly, the terminals of retinal ganglion cells in the kitten LGN have been examined following HRP injections in the eye at various ages, and it is apparent that the initial overlap of innervation derives at least in part from extra side 'twigs' in all layers of the ganglion (Sretavan & Shatz, 1986). Withdrawal of the side twigs occurs gradually in all but one layer, where there is considerable expansion of terminal branches.

Experiments similar to those performed on neonatal muscles indicate that the segregation into bands is dependent on a competition between terminals of the left and right eyes. If one eye is removed in the monkey embryo the terminals of the other eye in the cortex do not condense into bands (Rakic, 1981). Activity seems to be important, because if both eyes are sutured shut at birth the separation of the geniculate afferents into bands in layer IV is reduced (Swindale, 1981) and totally abolished if TTX is used to block spontaneous impulses arising in both eyes (Stryker & Harris, 1986). Separation of retinal ganglion cell afferents into eye-specific bands in the LGN is prevented by the absence of action potentials (Dubin, Stark &

Archer, 1986). Moreover, if only one eye is sutured shut at birth, its bands in layer IV shrink while those of the open eye remain wider than normal, suggesting that the more active open eye has a competitive advantage over the closed eye (Hubel *et al.*, 1977). The loss of terminal ramifications in the cortex from the less active geniculate neurons is reflected in the diminished size of their cell bodies. The cell bodies of the less active geniculate neurons shrink; however, this is an effect rather than a cause of the loss of the terminal branches, because cell bodies of neurons in the geniculate that do not share a cortical area with those of the other active eye do not shrink, nor is there cell shrinkage with binocular closure (Guillery, 1972, 1973). The loss of branches from inactive neurons is therefore a result of competition rather than non-specific withdrawal.

Further insight into the competitive interaction between the eyes has come from the experimental creation of alternating eye bands in the amphibian tectum. In amphibia the decussation of axons from each eye is complete, so there is normally no possibility of alternate banding of retinal afferents on the tectum. However, bands remarkably similar to those in the mammalian colliculus or visual cortex can be induced in the tectum if it receives projections from both eyes (Levine & Jacobson, 1975) or from a transplanted third eye (Law & Constantine-Paton, 1981); similar bands develop if a double nasal or double temporal compound eye projects to the tectum. It has been suggested that the bands develop when the normal guidance or recognition mechanism that distributes terminals across the target in a retinotopic fashion combines with some 'nearest neighbour' interaction between axons favouring local segregation of terminals from the same eye (Fawcett & Willshaw, 1982). Several observations implicate electrical activity in the interaction: one of the properties that neighbouring retinal ganglion cells share is relative synchrony of their activity; bands do not form in a tectum receiving projections from eyes rendered electrically silent with injections of tetrodotoxin (Meyer, 1982; Reh & Constantine-Paton, 1985); and the terminals vacate a small area of tectum that has been blocked postsynaptically with α-bungarotoxin and make new connections nearby (Freeman, 1977). The basis of the nearest neighbour interaction may therefore be synchronous activity in axon terminals and postsynaptic tectal cells, producing stabilisation of connections in localised bands. The randomised pattern of bands in the mammalian colliculus and cortex could develop in the same way, but in the LGN, where the bands are always in the same places, some additional guidance or recognition mechanism would seem to be needed.

Aberrant collaterals
Axons arising some distance from the normal region of terminal branching and often running to quite unusual destinations also exist in the developing CNS. The presence of these aberrant collaterals is inferred from the fact

that dyes injected into a given part of the brain of neonates can be detected subsequently in cell bodies at another site, whereas these cells are not labelled by an injection in the more mature animal. The axon collaterals that presumably pick up the dye are not removed by cell death, because the labelled cell bodies are still present weeks or months later. Thus an injection of dye into the pyramidal tract of newborn rats labels neurons right across the cortex, but in three week old rats injections do not label visual cortical neurons (Stanfield, O'Leary & Fricks, 1982). Similarly injections of dye into any part of the cortex of newborn rats label cells in the corresponding region of the contralateral cortex via collaterals in the corpus callosum, whereas in the adult the connections are restricted to somatosensory areas (O'Leary, Stanfield & Cowan, 1981) and to visual areas corresponding to the midline in visual space (Innocenti, 1981). A large proportion of the axons in the developing corpus callosum appear to be aberrant (Koppel & Innocenti, 1983). It is interesting that in cats with a natural or artificially induced squint, there are considerably more connections between the visual areas (Lund, Mitchell & Henry, 1978). This suggests that callosal collaterals joining areas that share the same region of visual space are retained because they are activated synchronously by visual stimuli.

Modification of receptive fields in the visual cortex

Visual information is delivered to the neurons of layer IV of the visual cortex by the geniculate afferents and is then distributed to the other layers by intracortical connections. The pattern of these connections and the changes that occur in them during development have not been visualised directly but have been inferred from the changes in the visual stimuli that activate the neurons, that is from changes in the receptive field properties of the neurons.

The knowledge of the properties of the neurons of the visual pathway is largely due to the work of Hubel and Wiesel, which will be summarised briefly here (for a review see Hubel & Wiesel, 1979, or Hubel, 1982). The receptive field of a neuron in the visual pathway is determined by the convergence of inputs from lower order neurons (fig. 9.6). Ganglion cells of the retina integrate the output of photoreceptors and respond to changes in light intensity in small circular patches of visual space. Neurons of the LGN and of layer IV have similar receptive fields and hence probably act mainly as relays for axons from the retina. Convergence is evident beyond layer IV, where neurons will usually respond only to stimuli with straight edges of a specific orientation moving in a specific small area of visual space. Neurons with similar orientation specificities are distributed across the cortex in regular columns (or more accurately 'slabs'). Neighbouring slabs have slightly different orientation preferences or specificities, so that in a direction normal to the slabs a full 360° of orientation specificities is encountered across a distance of several millimetres. Most neurons have

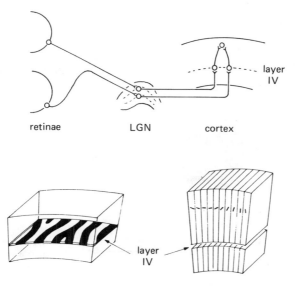

Fig. 9.6. Pattern of connections to the normal mammalian visual cortex. Above: convergence of inputs from each eye to produce binocular receptive fields in neurons beyond layer IV of the visual cortex. Convergence of many inputs produces the other receptive field properties of cortical neurons. LGN = lateral geniculate nucleus. Below left: pattern of banding of afferent from left and right eyes in layer IV. Below right: pattern of orientation slabs above and below layer IV.

inputs from both eyes and one of the interesting features of such binocular neurons is that the receptive field properties in each eye are identical. One eye usually dominates or drives a binocular neuron more effectively than the other and neurons with similar ocular dominance are organised in an independent pattern of columns that reflect the underlying bands of afferents in layer IV.

The binocular characteristics of cortical neurons were the first property found to be modifiable by experience (fig. 9.7). Hubel & Wiesel (1970) discovered that closing one eye of kittens for a few days or more during a 'critical period' of 4–8 weeks of age caused a marked reduction in the number of binocularly driven cells in the cortex. However, closure of one eye also causes shrinkage of its afferents in layer IV, so it was not clear whether the loss of binocularity of higher order neurons was a consequence of this shrinkage or a more direct effect on the intracortical connections. Loss of binocularity was also noted in cats that had been raised with an artificial squint (strabismus) following removal of one of the extraocular muscles, and the same effect was achieved when kittens were reared with daily alternate occlusion of each eye throughout the critical period (Hubel

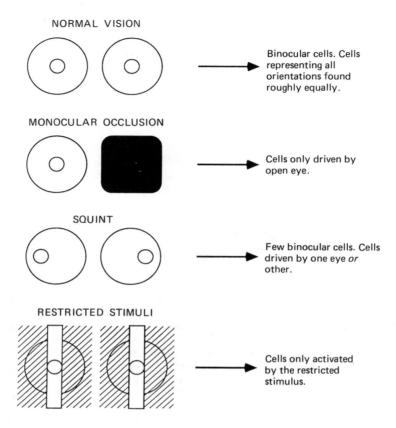

Fig. 9.7. Summary of effects of different visual experience on visual cortical cells during the 'critical period'.

& Wiesel, 1965). In both these cases there appeared to be no relative reduction in the cortical drive from either eye because the frequencies of purely monocular cells driven by each eye were usually similar. This meant that the loss of binocularity could be ascribed to a direct effect of the experimental manipulations on connections from the bands of layer IV that would normally converge to produce binocular neurons. The loss of binocularity is attributed to asynchrony of activity in adjacent bands, and this even applies to those animals with a squint: in a normal animal natural stimuli activate similar regions of each retina synchronously and hence adjacent afferent terminations in the cortex are synchronously active; in animals with a squint the synchronously active inputs from each eye are separated on the cortex, and adjacent bands are therefore asynchronous. A role for synchronous activity in the development of binocularly driven cells in the tectum of normal frogs was also proposed many years ago (Keating, 1974).

The orientation preference of cortical neurons has also been shown to be modified by experience. If kittens are reared with their vision restricted to contours of one orientation, then their cortical cells will respond only to contours of that orientation (Hirsch & Spinelli, 1971; Blakemore & Cooper, 1970; Stryker & Sherk, 1975; fig. 9.7). Again the modifications can be made only during a critical period of between four and eight weeks of age (e.g. Blakemore & Mitchell, 1973).

Given that abnormal visual experience can produce these changes in cortical circuitry, it is natural to ask whether normal visual experience plays some part in establishing normal response properties in cortical cells. The first observations of the properties of visual cortical neurons in normal young kittens gave the impression that all properties were innately determined (Hubel & Wiesel, 1963; Wiesel, 1982), which made their modifiability seem superfluous and potentially disadvantageous. However, it is now clear that the properties are only partly specified in visually naïve animals. In the kitten, receptive field sizes are larger than in the adult, orientation specificities are poorly defined or broadly tuned and in binocular cells there is poor concordance between the receptive field properties for each eye (Pettigrew, 1974). Dark rearing prevents much of the normal maturation of receptive field properties of cortical neurons, especially of binocular neurons (Fregnac & Imbert, 1984). In the monkey, some properties may be more accurately prespecified than in kittens (Wiesel & Hubel, 1974), but a rigorous study of spatial resolution and contrast sensitivity of cortical neurons in monkeys visually deprived since birth shows that these are much impaired (Blakemore & Vital Durand, 1983), and this is not due to a deterioration at the level of the lateral geniculate nucleus (Blakemore & Vital Durand, 1986). The critical period can therefore be seen as a time when cortical connections are easily modified and when the response properties resulting from the connections can be 'fine-tuned' by visual experience.

It is worth noting, however, that not all the improvements in visual performance are due to synaptic modifications at the cortical level or that they are confined to the critical period of up to eight weeks of age in kittens. Substantial improvements go on for up to four months after eye opening and at least some of the changes occur in the retina and in the eye itself (Teller & Movshon, 1986).

Mechanisms of the changes in cortical connections

It is clear from the previous sections that a major determinant of cortical connectivity is electrical activity and several other observations point to the importance of activity in the development of the cortex. In kittens deprived of all visual experience the responses of the neurons do not sharpen up, and the critical period is extended (Cynader & Mitchell, 1980). If deprivation is sufficiently prolonged, inputs from a deprived eye cease to have any functional connections in the cortex, suggesting that connections that are not reinforced by activity are permanently suppressed or withdrawn (Freeman & Ohzawa, 1988). If, on the other hand, vision is restricted to contours of a single orientation, then in the adult many more cells than normal respond specifically to that orientation, the orientation columns on the cortical surface are wider and there are few non-responsive cells (e.g. Rauschecker & Singer, 1981). Exposure to a single contour therefore rescues not only those neurons that would respond to that orientation in the normal adult, but also additional adjacent neurons. In the neonate these extra neurons would presumably be active in response to the stimulus because of the broad tuning of receptive fields.

Very little activity is needed to produce fine tuning of cortical neurons. Kittens reared in the dark need only be exposed to a restricted visual environment for an hour during the critical period to produce restricted responses in the cortical cells (Blakemore & Mitchell, 1973). Responses can even be specified in an anaesthetised visually naïve kitten in several minutes during the testing of a neuron's receptive field (Pettigrew, Olson & Barlow, 1973).

Competition between inputs is another major determinant of change in cortical connectivity. Competition is responsible for the development of discrete bands from each eye and of ocular dominance columns. Competition must also occur between inputs as cortical neurons develop orientation specificity: normal experience consists of exposure to contours of all possible orientations, but this does not maintain broad tuning of cortical cells, nor does it produce cells responding to several discrete orientations; instead, inputs to cortical cells compete until only one sharply tuned orientation succeeds in activating each cortical cell. A similar competition occurs between inputs from each eye, ensuring that the receptive field properties are identical in each eye.

A suitable mechanism invoking activity to achieve competition between inputs must involve a selective stabilisation of those inputs where there is synchrony of pre- and post-synaptic activity and a gradual loss of other inputs. Synapse modifications of this nature were suggested originally by Hebb (1949) to be the basis of learning and memory. Half a century later a key element in the mechanism may have been identified: N-methyl-D-aspartate (NMDA) receptors in the postsynaptic membrane. These receptors are known to be important in the phenomenon of Long-Term Potentiation (LTP) in another part of the cortex, the hippocampus (Chapter 10). Their involvement in the modification of connections in the visual cortex has now been demonstrated by two experiments: blockade of the receptors with a specific antagonist during monocular occlusion in kittens prevents the development of dominance by the open eye (Kleinschmidt, Bear & Singer, 1987), and iontophoretic application of NMDA agonists during presention of visual stimuli in kittens induces receptive fields specific to the stimulus (Greuel, Luhmann & Singer, 1988).

The NMDA receptor is activated by its endogenous ligand glutamate, but only if there is sufficient overall depolarisation of the cell (Chapter 10). This can explain why simultaneously active inputs may be stabilised, for the overall depolarisation will then be greater and each active input will assist others active at the same time. The degree of synchrony required in the timing of activity in convergent inputs to reinforce their connections is probably of the order of a few hundred milliseconds (see Von der Malsburg & Singer, 1988). This is quite a long time scale compared with that of conventional postsynaptic potentials but may be explicable because of the long lasting nature of dendritic responses. The need for adequate depolarisation if NMDA-coupled Ca^{2+} channels are to open can also explain why cortical plasticity can be blocked if non-specific excitatory noradrenergic (Kasamatsu & Pettigrew, 1976) and cholinergic (Bear & Singer, 1986) inputs are inactivated, for then the visual inputs on their own may not produce enough depolarisation. Similarly, the extra depolarisation produced by iontophoretic application of acetylcholine or noradrenaline can account for the observation of induction of receptive fields specific to visual stimuli paired with the iontophoresis (Greuel *et al.*, 1988).

Other critical periods

There are several examples of behavioural modification that may involve synaptic reorganisation in the auditory system. Adult barn owls are able to localise accurately sounds in space, but they lose this ability whenever binaural input is distorted with an earplug. Young birds, however, learn to compensate for an earplug (Knudsen, Knudsen & Esterly, 1982). Most song birds learn their songs during a restricted period in their first year of life. The learning involves modification of the bird's own innate calls until they match other adult calls or other environmental sounds (not necessarily even bird calls). After the critical period no new themes are acquired (Nottebohm, 1970). If sound patterns are excluded from the developing auditory system of neonatal mice by entraining all their primary auditory neurons to fire together, the cells in the inferior colliculus have tuning curves that are less sharply tuned than those of normal mice (Sanes & Constantine Paton, 1983).

Another example of neural modification that is produced only during a critical neonatal period concerns the development of the somatosensory cortex in rodents. In transverse sections of the cortex the normal adult animal has an array of characteristic barrel-shaped structures formed by the neurons associated with the sensory apparatus of a single facial vibrissa. Destruction of individual vibrissae in animals a few days old prevents the development of the corresponding barrels, whereas the same injury in the adult is without visible effect (Van der Loos & Woolsey, 1973). It is not clear whether this failure in barrel development is caused simply by the loss of afferent impulses to the cortex or by the degeneration of sensory and higher-order neurons following removal of the sensory target tissue.

The ability of animals to regulate their temperature is modified by experience during development. If the animals are not exposed to cool temperatures during rearing then their ability to maintain their body temperature in a cool environment is impaired (Cooper, Ferguson & Veale, 1980; Dawson *et al.*, 1982). This effect is not caused by changes in the sensitivity of peripheral thermoreceptors, so a central regulatory modification is likely.

In humans the critical period during which binocular vision can be compromised by strabismus extends up to approximately five years of age (Banks, Aslin & Letson, 1975). Beyond this age the excess connections responsible for binocularity in the visual cortex have presumably been eliminated.

Are there excess connections elsewhere in the cortex, and if so, what is the critical period for their modification? It is interesting to consider that in the first few years of life children can assimilate with little effort not just one but many languages and can develop skills in music and movement that are insuperably difficult for the inexperienced adult. Excess modifiable connections in appropriate regions of the cortex and elsewhere in the brain may be the basis of these remarkable feats of learning.

Conclusion
The essential feature of the stage of synapse reorganisation is that there are excess connections available from which a selection can be made, most likely by some kind of functional validation involving synchronous pre- and post-synaptic activity, possibly coupled with uptake of neuronal growth factors. The critical period probably corresponds to the time when excess connections are present and modifiable by experience-related neuronal activity. In the adult brain the excess connections that were not used during development are gone, but the mechanisms that led to the competition between the connections may still operate on the more limited connections that remain and thus contribute to adult plasticity.

Part 5

Adult plasticity

Chapter 10

The synaptic basis of learning

Introduction

It is widely held that the memory of an experience or the learning of a behaviour can occur only if there are stable changes in synaptic effectiveness. Indeed, it is difficult to imagine any other mechanism for memory and learning in the nervous systems of either vertebrates or invertebrates. This chapter deals with three model systems where synapses involved in learning have been identified and where progress is being made in describing the mechanisms responsible for the changes in synaptic effectiveness. In two of these systems (a reflex in the marine mollusc *Aplysia* and motor learning in the mammalian cerebellum) a stable behavioural change has been induced in the animal, a site of synaptic change has been identified and underlying mechanisms are being analysed. In *Aplysia* there is now a detailed knowledge of the biochemical mechanisms involved, but in the cerebellum there is still much to learn about these. In the third system (long-term potentiation in the hippocampus) neuronal connections are modified by activity delivered through stimulating electrodes. This approach offers the advantage that synaptic modification is more easily studied, and much has now been learned about subcellular mechanisms; however, the application to specific instances of learning in the animal is less direct.

Modification of a reflex in *Aplysia*

Invertebrates display stable, adaptive changes in their behaviour, and their nervous systems have far fewer nerve cells than vertebrates, so they are an obvious starting point for investigating the neuronal basis of learning. The gill withdrawal reflex of the marine mollusc *Aplysia californica* (the sea hare) is a behaviour that exhibits stable long-term changes and it has been chosen by Kandel and his collaborators for investigation (Kandel & Schwartz, 1982). The reflex is monosynaptic and consists of a brief defensive withdrawal of gills and siphon evoked by light tactile or electrical stimulation of the siphon (fig. 10.1).

Repeated stimulation of the siphon causes a reduction of the withdrawal response that can last for up to several weeks. This is the phenomenon of *habituation*, the simplest form of learning. Strong electrical shocks to the

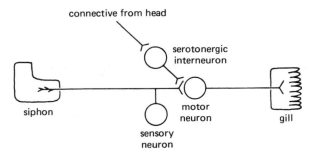

Fig. 10.1. Pathways for sensitisation of gill withdrawal reflex in *Aplysia* (after Kandel & Schwartz, 1982.)

head (which themselves produce massive withdrawal responses) cause an immediate and long lasting enhancement, or *sensitisation*, of the gill withdrawal reflex. Habituation and sensitisation are examples of *non-associative* learning. In the first case activation of the reflex-inducing pathway on its own changes its efficacy and in the second, the siphon-gill withdrawal pathway does not have to be active for the modification to occur. A shock to the tail can also cause some sensitisation of the gill withdrawal reflex, but more importantly, if a touch to the siphon is *paired* with the tail shock about 15 times, then there is a marked additional enhancement of the withdrawal to siphon touch alone which lasts for several weeks (Carew, Walters & Kandel, 1981). This shows that *associative learning* or *classical conditioning* of the withdrawal response has occurred, with the marked response to tail shock (the unconditioned stimulus) becoming associated with the siphon touch alone (the conditioned stimulus).

Habituation is due to depression of transmission at the synapse between the sensory terminals and motor neurons. The depression is presynaptic and due to a fall in the number of Ca^{2+} channels in the presynaptic terminal. This is possibly caused by the rise in intracellular Ca^{2+} ion concentration in the terminals following repeated activation of the pathway (Klein, Shapiro & Kandel, 1980). With fewer functioning Ca^{2+} channels, less calcium enters per nerve impulse and so less transmitter is released.

The basis of sensitisation has now also been largely established. Enhancement of the withdrawal response is found to be caused by increased release of transmitter from the terminals of the sensory neurons. Activity in axons in the connectives running from the head region to the abdominal ganglion is thought to bring about this increase in release by a mechanism of *presynaptic facilitation* mediated by serotonin (5-hydroxytryptamine) released from interneurons onto the sensory nerve's synapses on motor neurons. The evidence for this is as follows: serotonin applied artificially to the sensory neurons produces a similar enhancement of transmission

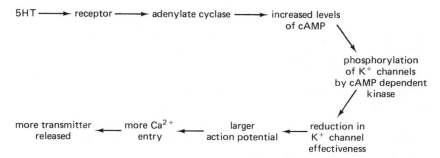

Fig. 10.2. Sequence of events in sensory terminals leading to presynaptic facilitation in *Aplysia*.

(Castellucci & Kandel, 1976; Brunelli, Castellucci & Kandel, 1976); a group of interneurons in the ganglion activated by head connectives (the L29 cells) produce a long-lasting facilitation of transmitter release if they are stimulated (Hawkins, Castellucci & Kandel, 1981), and these cells have all the morphological properties of serotonergic neurons; finally, contacts between these neurons, labelled with ^{3}H-serotonin, and sensory neurons labelled with HRP, were demonstrated in EM autoradiographs of the ganglion neuropil (Bailey *et al.*, 1981). Serotonin produces its effects on the sensory neuron terminals by activating adenylate cyclase and thus increasing their intracellular concentration of cyclic AMP. Potassium channels are then phosphorylated via a cyclic AMP-dependent protein kinase, and this causes a reduction in the number of effective K^+ channels in the membrane, which in turn allows a greater influx of Ca^{2+} during the sensory nerve terminal depolarisations and hence a greater release of transmitter (Kandel & Schwartz, 1982); see fig. 10.2.

More recently it has proved possible to reconstitute circuits between isolated sensory neurons and motor neurons in culture and to mimic the action of presynaptic facilitatory pathways with bath-applied serotonin (Montarolo *et al.*, 1986). Brief single applications of serotonin generate a short term facilitation which is not sensitive to inhibitors of protein or RNA synthesis, but repeated application of serotonin produces long-term facilitation which is blocked by the inhibitors of synthesis but only if used while serotonin is in the culture. Thus short-term facilitation may modify existing structures in the sensory terminals, such as the K^+ channels, but longer term events may need new structures. Further biochemical comparison of long-term-facilitated and non-facilitated sensory neurons shows that the amounts of two proteins are specifically increased during facilitation (Barzilai *et al.*, 1989). Long term retention of sensitisation *in vivo* is accompanied by increases in the number of varicosities that each sensory terminal makes on a motor neuron (Bailey & Chen, 1989).

Recently, a possible molecular explanation of the classical conditioning of the withdrawal reflex has been proposed (Abrams & Kandel, 1988). The adenylate cyclase responsible for presynaptic facilitation by serotonin is also sensitive to calcium-calmodulin. When Ca^{2+} enters the sensory terminal during an action potential at the same time as serotonin receptors are activated, two stimulatory effectors (Ca^{2+} and serotonin) will then converge on the adenylate cyclase. In this way more cAMP might be generated than by either input alone. It is unlikely, however, that only presynaptic changes occur during associative learning. There is evidence that the synapses between motor neurons and the gill musculature are also facilitated (Lukowiak & Colebrook, 1988).

Motor learning in the cerebellum

Evidence of various kinds implicates the cerebellum in the control of movement. Anatomical and physiological studies have shown that the cerebellum has afferent and efferent connections with other brain structures involved in the initiation and execution of movement and that it also receives a wide range of sensory inputs. Focal stimulation of discrete areas of cerebellar cortex produces movements and cerebellar lesions produce marked defects in movement co-ordination (ataxia). A closer analysis of the effects of cerebellar lesions shows that they produce defects in the retention and acquisition of learned movements. In cats, for example, eyelid blinking elicited by a puff of air directed at one eye can be conditioned to occur in response to an acoustic stimulus and ablation of the ipsilateral cerebellar hemisphere selectively abolishes the conditioned response without affecting the blinking reflex; moreover the conditioned response cannot be acquired following hemicerebellectomy (Lincoln, McCormick & Thompson, 1982).

When the details of circuitry in the cerebellar cortex were worked out by J. C. Eccles and others (see fig. 10.3), there was much speculation about how motor learning might be achieved in the cerebellum. The models proposed are all very similar (Marr, 1969; Albus, 1971; Gilbert, 1974). It is assumed that activity in Purkinje cells produces specific 'elemental' movements. Each Purkinje cell receives a strong input from a single climbing fibre, which may be closely connected with the sensory receptors associated with the Purkinje cell's specific movement, or with the cortical area where the movement is initiated. The Purkinje cells also receive weaker inputs from a wide range of sensory receptors via the parallel fibres of the granule cells, which are connected to the mossy fibre inputs to the cerebellum. Activity in the climbing fibre was envisaged by Marr as somehow increasing the efficacy of any parallel fibre–Purkinje cell synapses that were also active at the same time (fig. 10.3). In the above example of conditioned eyelid blinking, the puff of air would produce activity in the climbing fibres that synapse on Purkinje cells associated with eyelid movement, the acoustic stimulus would produce activity in parallel fibres and transmission at the

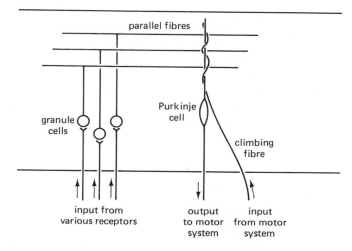

Fig. 10.3 Motor learning in the cerebellar cortex. Synchronous activity in a climbing fibre and a parallel fibre is thought to modify the strength of the synapse of the parallel fibre on the Purkinje cell.

synapses of the parallel fibres on the eyelid Purkinje cells would be stably enhanced because of the synchrony between parallel fibres and climbing fibres. Conditioning would be achieved when the acoustic stimulus alone could excite the Purkinje cells via the parallel fibres and thereby elicit the blink.

Albus (1971) produced a similar theory, but reasoned that the system would be more efficient and inherently more stable if transmission at the parallel fibre–Purkinje cell synapses were made *less* effective by conjoint activity in the climbing fibres. Experiments performed to test the interaction between the climbing and parallel fibres on the Purkinje cells support the Albus theory (Andersen, 1982). In a study on conscious monkeys that were learning a hand movement, parallel fibre-induced activity was assayed in Purkinje cells as simple spikes and climbing fibre-induced activity was assayed in the same cells as complex spikes (the climbing fibre input is more powerful than the parallel fibre input). In the arm area of the cerebellum Purkinje cells were found in which there were transient increases in complex spike activity during the learning period and in these cells there was a decrease in simple spike activity that persisted after the complex spike activity had returned to normal (Gilbert & Thach, 1977). In an elegant study by Ito and his coworkers parallel fibres in the vestibular cerebellum were stimulated via the ipsilateral vestibular nerve, climbing fibres were stimulated where they originate in the inferior olive and activity was recorded in Purkinje cells. Conjoint stimulation of parallel and climbing fibres was followed by a depression in parallel fibre synaptic transmission that lasted in some cases as long as the recording from the Purkinje cell could be maintained (up to one hour). Transmission from the unstimulated contralateral vestibular nerve was unaffected and random stimulation of parallel and climbing fibres did not produce changes in parallel fibre synaptic transmission. Stimulation of climbing fibres and conjoint ionto-phoretic application of glutamate, the presumed transmitter at the parallel fibres synapses, led to a decreased sensitivity of the Purkinje cells to the transmitter. This is strong evidence that the change in transmission of the parallel fibre synapses is postsynaptic in origin. One possible mechanism is a desensitisation of any glutamate receptors activated during the period of high intradendritic Ca^{2+} concentration following climbing fibre stimula-tion (Ito, Sakurai & Tongroach, 1982).

Long-term potentiation in the hippocampus

The hippocampus is the phylogenetically old part of the cerebral cortex connected with the limbic system. There is considerable evidence that the hippocampus is important in acquiring and retaining some forms of learning. Damage to the hippocampus is known to produce deficits in memory in humans. Rats also lose the memory of how best to use a maze to get a food reward following hippocampal lesions, and cannot relearn (Olton, Walker & Gage, 1978). Moreover a high proportion of the neurons in the hippocampus in conscious rats show alterations in their firing patterns that are specific to the animal's position in a familar environment (O'Keefe & Dostrovsky, 1971; O'Keefe, 1976).

Synaptic transmission in the hippocampus was first studied in anaesthe-tised rabbits in response to direct stimulation of one of its main afferent tracts, the perforant path (Bliss & Lømo, 1973) (fig. 10.4). The perforant path arises in the entorhinal cortex and terminates on dendrites of the granule cells of the dentate area of the hippocampus. The excitatory postsynaptic potential evoked in the granule cells by perforant path stimulation can be recorded with an extracellular electrode as a synaptic wave caused by the flow of current into the dendrites. With sufficient stimulation there can also be a superimposed spike caused by the synchro-nous firing of an action potential in some granule cells. Single stimuli to the perforant path every few seconds produce a constant postsynaptic activa-tion of the granule cells, but if an extra train of stimuli at a frequency of 10–100 Hz is applied for 10 or more seconds, substantial short and long-term changes in transmission occur. During the train there is a potentiation of transmission, as shown by increases in wave and spike amplitude and a decrease in spike latency. Immediately after the train there is a period of depression lasting for up to a minute, but thereafter there is a return of potentiation that can last for hours in anaesthetised animals and for over a week in conscious animals. This latter phenomenon has been called long-term potentiation (LTP) and it has been observed in several other pathways

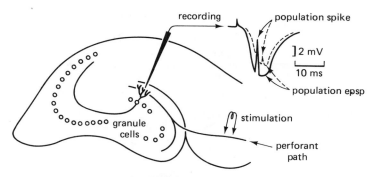

Fig. 10.4. Long-term potentiation (LTP) of evoked responses in dendritic layer of dentate area of hippocampus following stimulation of the perforant path. Dashed and continuous lines in trace represent responses to single stimuli before and after LTP respectively. epsp = excitatory postsynaptic potential (after Bliss & Lømo, 1973).

within the hippocampus. Elsewhere in the nervous system potentiation can be produced by trains of stimuli, but in all cases high frequencies and long trains are required to produce the effect and the potentiation lasts only for minutes or at most hours.

LTP does not normally occur unless a sufficient number of axons is activated by the conditioning train of stimuli. This implies that there is some kind of co-operative interaction between axons on the postsynaptic cells. However, where two separate pathways that can both be potentiated converge on the same cells, LTP of one pathway causes only a short term depression in the other and does not affect its potentiation and this applies even where both pathways converge on the same general region of the dendrites (Dunwiddie & Lynch, 1978). This suggests that LTP induction requires presynaptic firing to be coincident with adequate depolarisation of the postsynaptic membrane. Consistent with this suggestion are the observations that single presynaptic volleys cause LTP if the postsynaptic cell is artificially depolarised with an intracellular electrode, and that hyperpolarisation of the cell prevents LTP (Gustafsson & Wigstrom, 1988).

Some progress has been made in discovering the biochemical sequelae of simultaneous presynaptic activity and postsynaptic depolarisation (fig. 10.5). A key element may be the unique properties of the NMDA receptor (cf. pp.104–5). This receptor is activated by the synthetic compound N-methyl-D-aspartate and the naturally-occurring excitatory transmitter glutamate. Binding of glutamate does not open the calcium ionophore associated with the receptor unless the postsynaptic membrane is also sufficiently depolarised (this removes blocking Mg^{2+} ions from the channel). Calcium ions then enter and start a train of intermediate steps that enhance subsequent transmission. Use of selective blockers of NMDA and

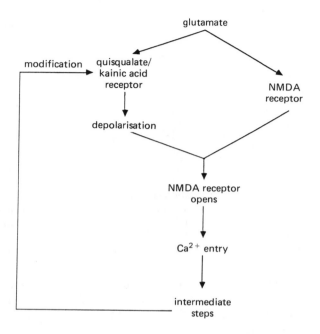

Fig. 10.5. Possible mechanism of induction of LTP. Release of sufficient transmitter (glutamate) produces depolarisation and activation of NMDA receptor, which leads via a Ca^{2+}-dependent step to permanent modification (increased sensitivity) of quisqualate-kainic acid receptors.

other receptors for glutamate (quisqualate–kainic acid receptors) has shown that while NMDA receptors have to be activated if LTP is to occur, only the other glutamate-sensitive receptors are modified (Kauer, Malenka & Nicoll, 1988; Muller, Joly & Lynch, 1988). The nature of the intermediate changes leading to receptor modification or other possible postsynaptic changes that might contribute to improved transmission are still debatable. There is evidence for the involvement of both a calcium/calmodulin-dependent kinase and protein kinase C (T.H. Brown *et al.*, 1988; Anwyl, 1989; Malenka *et al.*, 1989).

Structural changes have been reported in the hippocampus following LTP induction. Fifkova & Van Harreveld (1977) performed an electron microscopic analysis of the dentate area following perforant pathway stimulation and found a significant increase in dendrite spine diameters only in the region of perforant path termination. A more recent analysis has also detected significant changes in spine diameters and lengths after LTP (Andersen *et al.*, 1987). An increased conductance between the dendritic spine synapses and the dendritic shaft might accompany this structural change and this could increase the postsynaptic effect of synapses on those spines. GAP-43, a protein found in growing axons (Skene, 1989), and protein kinase C, which is known to phosphorylate it, are both present in high concentrations in the hippocampus (Nelson *et al.*, 1989); they might be involved in producing the long-term structural changes.

Presynaptic changes may also be important in the maintenance of LTP. It has been found that a perfusate of the dentate area contains more glutamate ions following potentiation of the perforant path (Dolphin, Errington & Bliss, 1982). In hippocampal slices pertussis toxin, a blocker of G protein activation, prevents LTP development at a presynaptic site (Goh & Pennefather, 1989) and there is also evidence that the inositol/IP3 second messenger system is activated in hippocampal synaptosomes following LTP induction (Lynch *et al.*, 1988). This might provide increased Ca^{2+} concentrations inside the presynaptic terminals, thus boosting transmitter output. The presynaptic changes responsible for greater transmitter output may not be generated independently of the postsynaptic changes, for no LTP is present following NMDA receptor block (Collingridge & Bliss, 1987).

The relevance of LTP to learning in the intact animal and of the NMDA receptor in the process has been strengthened by examining the effect of a specific NMDA blocker, AP5, on learning in rats (Morris *et al.*, 1986). Intraventricular infusion of AP5 selectively impaired the ability to learn spatial cues.

Chapter 11

Nerve injury, degeneration and trophic effects

Introduction

A striking feature of nerve cells and the cells that they innervate in the periphery is that their normal morphology, biochemistry and physiology are dependent on their synaptic connections. The first evidence for this was the observation that denervated limbs became wasted and that the healthy state of the limb tissues was restored only following successful reinnervation. Closer examination of denervated target cells shows that they undergo marked changes in many of their properties. It is apparent, therefore, that normal target cell properties are maintained in some way by the nerve. This influence of the nerve on its target is called the orthograde trophic effect. Orthograde trophic effects could be mediated either by postsynaptic electrical activity evoked by the nerve or by substances synthesised in the nerve cell body, transported along the axons and released onto the target cells (fig. 11.1). In mammalian skeletal muscle, the trophic effect is found to be mediated predominantly by the muscle fibre action potentials. Substances released by the motor nerves might be expected to have little or no effect on most muscle properties because of the relatively small size and localised distribution of the nerve terminals in relation to the bulk of the muscle. However, properties of the synaptic region of the muscle fibres are probably influenced directly by neurotransmitter or other nerve-released substances, and other innervated tissues and glial cells appear to be maintained by trophic substances released by nerves.

Effects of axotomy are not restricted to cells distal to the site of injury. Neurons that have been disconnected from their targets also undergo characteristic morphological changes that have been termed 'chromatolysis' and there are accompanying changes in physiological and biochemical properties of the neurons, changes in the satellite cells, and changes in synaptic connections. There is considerable evidence that these retrograde changes are mediated at least partly by the interruption of the retrograde transport of a trophic factor that is released by target tissues and probably also by glial cells, and that is taken up by the axons (fig. 11.1). Nerve Growth Factor appears to be a trophic factor for sympathetic and sensory nerves, and evidence for the existence of other factors that are effective on other neurons is beginning to accumulate.

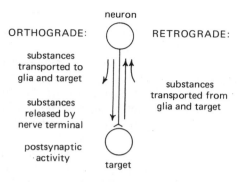

Fig. 11.1. Orthograde and retrograde trophic influences between neuron, glia and target cells. Compare fig. 8.4.

The properties that the nerve, target and glial cells develop after they have been disconnected from each other are not simply degenerative: in many respects the new properties are similar to those of embryonic cells. The changes are therefore appropriate for encouraging the regrowth of axons, the re-establishment of connections, and finally the redevelopment of the normal, differentiated adult state.

Orthograde trophic effects on peripheral nerve

A special (and obvious) case of trophic dependence is that of a nerve cell's own extremities. The axon contains no machinery to manufacture the large number of proteins that it contains, so when isolated from its cell body by nerve section or crush it is fated eventually to degenerate. The earliest changes in the distal nerve stump of a motor neuron after it has been separated from the cell body by axotomy occur at the neuromuscular junction. Failure of the spontaneous and evoked release of transmitter occurs first, accompanied by disruption of the nerve terminal. Failure is delayed if the nerve is transected further away from the muscle, and the signal for failure appears to travel distally from the site of nerve transection at a rate of about 1 cm per hour in mammals (Miledi & Slater, 1970), which is the rate of fast axoplasmic transport. The changes are probably initiated by a drop in the level of some substance supplied by the cell body rather than by the entry of substances into the axon at the site of injury because the proximal stump of the axon still connected to the cell body does not usually degenerate.

Degeneration spreads backwards from the terminals (Brown, Hopkins & Keynes, 1982a; Lunn, Brown & Perry, 1990). The reasons for this are unclear but it may be because the terminals are more accessible to invading macrophages and other white blood cells. These cells play more than a simple scavenging role in the process of degeneration; if their recruitment is prevented or is absent, as is the case in a mutant strain of mouse, then axonal degeneration is extremely slow, taking weeks rather than hours or days to occur (Lunn *et al.*, 1989). It seems that loss of trophic support leads to changes in the axon that are not immediately critical for function but are detected by Schwann cells or resident macrophages. These in turn recruit the circulating macrophages and other leukocytes that secrete agents hastening the degeneration of trophically deprived axons. The Schwann cells respond to the changes in the axon by retracting from nodes of Ranvier and extruding their own myelin into the space outside their basal lamina (Crang & Blakemore, 1986). The breakdown and removal of the myelin and the mitosis of the Schwann cells that follow are also dependent on invasion of the nerve by macrophages (Beuche & Friede, 1984). There is recent evidence that transforming growth factors $\beta 1$ and $\beta 2$, which can be produced by macrophages, are mitogens for Schwann cells (Ridley *et al.*, 1989). The result of all these changes is large numbers of dedifferentiated Schwann cells lying within their basal lamina sheaths, forming the so-called bands of Büngner, which provide an ideal pathway for regrowing axons (see Chapter 12). For example, one product of activated macrophages is Interleukin-1 and this stimulates the production of Nerve Growth Factor by Schwann cells (Lindholm *et al.*, 1987), which may be necessary for afferent nerve fibre regeneration (Johnson, Taniuchi & Di Stefano, 1988). If axons do not manage to reinnervate the distal stump, Schwann cells themselves gradually atrophy and eventually degenerate (Weinberg & Spencer, 1978).

The nature of the signals passing between axons and Schwann cells remains unclear. Labelled proteins transported down the axon from the cell body do not appear to cross into the Schwann cells, although some membrane components do (Droz, 1979). Physical transfer of material may not even be necessary if the trophic effect is mediated by contact between the Schwann cell and a component of the axon membrane.

Orthograde trophic effects on mammalian skeletal muscle

The major changes that have been identified in muscle cells following denervation are summarised in fig. 11.2. They include a small depolarisation of the resting potential, changes in contractile properties, changes in junctional and extrajunctional membrane properties, changes in basal lamina composition and atrophy of fibres. One other major change in muscle is, of course, the lack of action potentials and it is now clear that the loss of activity is responsible for most of the changes in muscle properties following denervation. In the experiment that first showed this conclusively, extrajunctional acetylcholine sensitivity was assayed in muscles that were denervated but stimulated directly through electrodes implanted next to the muscles. It was found that increases in sensitivity associated with denervation did not occur in the stimulated muscles, whereas muscles with intact nerves in which activity had been blocked with small cuffs containing

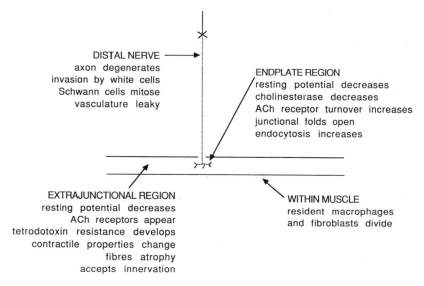

Fig. 11.2. Changes in peripheral nerve and muscle which are caused directly or indirectly by loss of orthograde trophic influences following axotomy. ACh = acetylcholine.

local anaesthetic developed changes characteristic of the denervated state (Lømo & Rosenthal, 1972). Other extrajunctional membrane properties and junctional cholinesterase are also maintained by activity (e.g. Westgaard, 1975; Weinberg & Hall, 1979).

It has been known for some time that extensive changes in the contractile properties of skeletal muscles occur after exchanging nerves between 'slow' muscles (composed mostly of slow (type I) motor units) and 'fast' muscles (composed mostly of fast (type II) motor units), even if this is done in adult animals (Buller, Eccles & Eccles, 1960). It has since been shown that these changes can be brought about by an appropriate pattern of electrical activity delivered through electrodes either to denervated muscles (Lømo, Westgaard & Dahl, 1974) or to muscles with their nerves intact (Salmons & Sreter, 1976). Thus continuous low frequency activation (a pattern of firing characteristic of motor neurons innervating slow oxidative motor units) slows the contraction time of fast glycolytic muscles and causes them to develop more mitochondria and capillaries. On the other hand, the same number of impulses delivered in intermittent high-frequency bursts (a pattern characteristic of fast, fatiguable motor units) 'converts' slow muscles into fast muscles, changing both myofibrillar and excitation–contraction coupling proteins. This control of a muscle's contractile characteristics by pattern of its use is an eminently sensible, adaptive strategy.

The basis for the changes in properties is synthesis of different isoforms of the protein subunits that are used in the construction of myosin, tropomyosin and troponin (Pette & Staron, 1988). The conversion from slow to fast properties is not perfect, because slow isoforms continue to be synthesised and the newly synthesised fast isoforms are not identical to those of a true fast muscle (Gorza *et al.*, 1988). Thus, it does not seem possible to make a fibre that has been developmentally determined to be slow (Miller & Stockdale, 1986, 1987) identical to a developmentally determined fast fibre. Each intrinsic type has, however, an adaptive range (Westgaard & Lømo, 1988) of variable magnitude (slow fibres having a larger range than fast) so that considerable overlap of properties between the basic types can be achieved by the appropriate pattern of stimulation. The intracellular mechanism of the control by pattern of activity is uncertain.

Is there nevertheless an additional trophic effect, independent of muscle activity, mediated by substances released by the nerve? Several different experimental approaches have been taken to try to answer this question.

Effects of blockade of axonal transport

Colchicine applied locally to peripheral nerves inhibits axonal transport and eventually causes nerve degeneration, presumably through depletion of trophic substances in the distal portion of the nerve. Denervation-like changes develop in muscles when their nerves are treated with colchicine, and this occurs before the nerves degenerate and cease to activate the muscle. It was thought at first that these changes could be attributed to reduced release of a trophic agent, but this is made unlikely by the observation that colchicine causes similar changes directly when it reaches the muscle fibres via the circulation (Lømo, 1974).

Effects of blockade of activity

If nerve conduction or synaptic transmission is blocked leaving the nerve otherwise intact, many denervation-like changes in the inactive muscle are found to be less well developed than in fully denervated muscles. However, it cannot be concluded that intact, but inactive, nerves have a residual trophic effect on muscle properties: the changes seen with denervation are caused in part by the processes associated with degeneration of the cut axons (Jones & Vrbova, 1974; Lømo & Westgaard, 1976; Cangiano & Lutzemberger, 1980; Cangiano, 1985), and denervated muscles also contain large numbers of dividing fibroblasts and other cell types (Murray & Robbins, 1982*a,b*) that may produce effects on muscle. For example, Tumour Necrosis Factor, a product of activated macrophages, is known to cause depolarisation of skeletal muscle fibres (Tracey *et al.*, 1986). Attempts have been made to prolong blockade to allow comparisons with long term denervation when the effects of nerve degeneration might have subsided, but where differences between blocked and denervated muscles persist it cannot be guaranteed that all nerve-evoked activity in the paralysed muscles has been prevented. Complete blockade with botulinum toxin *can* produce convergence of properties in blocked and denervated muscles of mice (Brown, Hopkins & Keynes, 1982*b*), but the toxin may also prevent release of any putative trophic factor. These experiments therefore remain inconclusive.

Effects of nerve-derived substances on muscles in vitro
Cultures of embryonic muscles provide a convenient system to analyse nerve-derived substances which might promote synaptogenesis (Chapter 7). In a similar way organ cultures of muscles have also been used to determine whether such substances can inhibit or reverse denervation-induced changes. A protein extracted from chicken sciatic nerves can induce morphological maturation in cultured embryonic muscle (Markelonis & Oh, 1979). This protein, originally called sciatin, was found to be identical to transferrin. Extracts of various tissues, including nerve, can stimulate the synthesis of cholinesterase at the endplate of organ-cultured muscles (Davey, Younkin & Younkin, 1979), and an extract of spinal cord can alter properties of the action potential and the acetylcholine receptors of denervated muscles towards those of the innervated state (Kuromi, Gonoi & Hosegawa, 1979). Whether motor nerves release enough of these substances to exert a trophic effect *in vivo* remains to be seen. This qualification also applies to the trophic effect demonstrated by another nerve extract applied daily to denervated rat muscles *in vivo* (Davis & Heinicke, 1984).

Short-term organ cultures of muscles have also been used to investigate the fall in resting potential that occurs following denervation (Albuquerque, Schuh & Kauffman, 1971). Changes were delayed in the muscles with longer nerve stumps, but these experiments do not distinguish between the effects of loss of a putative trophic factor and the direct effects of degeneration associated with denervation (discussed above), both of which would be delayed by a longer stump length.

Orthograde trophic effects in other tissues

Neurons
In experiments performed earlier this century, assays of end organ responses to intravenous infusions of neurotransmitters demonstrated that denervated (i.e. decentralised) sympathetic ganglia developed supersensitivity to acetylcholine following denervation. At least some of this rise in sensitivity to transmitter in sympathetic ganglia is caused not by an increase in numbers of postsynaptic receptors but by a decrease in cholinesterase activity (Dunn & Marshall, 1985). However, supersensitivity in denervated parasympathetic ganglion cells in the heart has been detected by recording intracellular responses to iontophoretically applied acetylcholine (Kuffler,

Dennis & Harris, 1971) and so is of postsynaptic origin like that in skeletal muscle. If the preganglionic nerve is allowed to regenerate into the cardiac ganglion this sensitivity is reduced in many ganglion cells before activity can be evoked in them by nerve stimulation, suggesting that a trophic agent independent of postsynaptic activity is responsible for maintaining the normal sensitivity (Dennis & Sargent, 1979).

The regulation of the enzyme tyrosine hydroxylase in the superior cervical ganglion has received considerable attention. Section of the preganglionic input to the ganglion in the adult produces a gradual decline in the level of tyrosine hydroxylase (Hendry, Iversen & Black, 1973), suggesting that it is under trophic control by the preganglionic nerves. Activity in the *presynaptic* terminals appears to have the important regulatory influence, because a brief period of intense preganglionic stimulation produces a significant increase in tyrosine hydroxylase activity in the ganglion three days later, whereas the same stimulation applied to the ganglion cells via the postsynaptic nerve is ineffective (Chalazonitis & Zigmond, 1980). The effect of presynaptic stimulation is antagonised by the ganglion blocking drug hexamethonium, suggesting that the responsible agent could be the transmitter itself (Chalazonitis & Zigmond, 1980). There are two mechanisms by which tyrosine hydroxylase activity is increased. The first involves phosphorylation of pre-existing enzyme. This is rapid in action and can be induced by a variety of peptide and other transmitters acting via several protein kinases (Zigmond, Schwarzschild & Rittenhouse, 1989). A slower mechanism occurs over a period of days by means of an increase of mRNA for tyrosine hydroxylase (Black, Chikaraishi & Lewis, 1985).

The transmitter noradrenaline in the postganglionic nerves also appears to be the trophic agent responsible for maintenance of the pineal gland. Denervation of the pineal, or simply a period of relative inactivity, produces supersensitivity to noradrenaline, whereas presynaptic activity reduces the sensitivity and increases synthesis of the enzyme that produces melatonin in the gland. Noradrenaline probably mediates these effects by hyperpolarising the gland cells (Zigmond & Bowers, 1981).

In the CNS, denervation (deafferentation) can lead to cell shrinkage and even death of the postsynaptic neurons. For example, cells in the lateral geniculate nucleus degenerate when the optic nerve is cut in monkeys, even in adults (Matthews, Cowan & Powell, 1960). Activity is at least partly responsible for maintaining these cells, because closure of one eye leads to cell shrinkage (Hubel & Wiesel, 1963).

Frog slow muscle
Some muscles in the frog do not normally have an action potential, but instead are depolarised entirely by acetylcholine released from terminals distributed along the fibres. An action potential mechanism does develop on denervated fibres, and it is suppressed when the nerve regenerates

(Schmidt & Stefani, 1977). Paralysis with α-bungarotoxin also induces the action potential mechanism, which indicates that acetylcholine itself is likely to be the agent that maintains the normal non-excitable state of the muscle, possibly via the depolarisation it causes (Miledi & Uchitel, 1981).

Sensory end-organs

Sensory neurons also exert trophic effects on their end-organs. Taste buds, for example, atrophy rapidly following section of the gustatory nerves and return to normal following reinnervation. The maintenance is to some extent non-specific, in that non-gustatory sensory nerves will reinstate the function of the end-organ, whereas motor nerves will not (Zalewski, 1969). However, little more is known about the nature of this trophic support. Calcitonin-gene-related peptide released from sensory cells of the olfactory epithelium has the capacity to make periglomerular cells of the olfactory bulb become dopaminergic (Denis-Donini, 1989), raising the possibility that peptide or other transmitter substances released by sensory nerves at central terminals are also released in the periphery and maintain end-organs.

Effects of nerves on limb regeneration

One well known trophic action of nerves is their ability to support the regrowth of amputated limbs in urodeles and crustacea. It seems that this action is non-specific, depending on quantity rather than type of nerves (see review by Singer, 1974). The regrowth of the amputated limb is due to mitosis of mesenchymal cells at the stump tip, and this mitosis is stimulated by a glial growth factor (Brockes & Kintner, 1986; see Chapter 4).

Invertebrate trophic effects

There have been a few isolated observations of trophic effects in invertebrates. The peripheral stump of a severed nerve degenerates, but in some cases the degeneration is very slow (action potentials can be conducted for several months) and the severed ends can fuse together again (Hoy, Bittner & Kennedy, 1967). Crustacean leg muscles atrophy following denervation but do not develop supersensitivity to the excitatory transmitter glutamate (Frank, 1974). A small increase in sensitivity can be detected in denervated insect leg muscles (Usherwood, 1969). Activity is important for transforming a particular fast muscle into a slow muscle in lobsters during development (Govind & Kent, 1982), and it is probably also important for maintaining muscle properties in the adult. The pattern of activity also determines the different properties of motor neurons innervating the crusher and cutter claws in lobsters (Luenicka, Blundon & Govind, 1988).

Retrograde trophic effects

The most obvious structural change in neurons that have been disconnected from their periphery is dispersion of the aggregates of ribosomes and endoplasmic reticulum in the cell body. This was first observed last century in the light microscope as a dissolution of the Nissl substance, and the term chromatolysis was coined to describe it. Other structural changes were detected with the light microscope, and a proportion of cells was also seen to die. A wide variety of techniques has since been used to analyse the chromatolytic changes that occur in and around axotomised neurons. These changes are summarised in fig. 11.3. Biophysical and biochemical investigations have revealed transient increases in RNA and protein synthesis and turnover rates not only in the nerve cell body but also in the surrounding glial cells, some of which divide (Watson, 1974). An early increase in metabolic activity can be detected autoradiographically following the uptake and accumulation of 2-deoxyglucose in axotomised neurons (Singer & Mehler, 1980). The synthesis of actin, the embryonic $T\alpha$-1 subunit of tubulin and GAP-43 all rise over the course of a week (Skene, 1989; Tetzlaff *et al.*, 1988) the first changes being detectable within a few hours of axotomy using *in situ* hybridisation techniques for mRNA (Miller *et al.*, 1989). At the same time synthesis of neurofilament proteins falls (Tetzlaff *et al.*, 1988). Physiological techniques show alterations in the action potential waveform recorded in the cell body and a loss of presynaptic drive, which in the electron microscope correlates with the shedding of synaptic boutons, involution of the postsynaptic membrane and retraction of dendrites (e.g. Purves, 1975).

The first attempts to identify the cause of chromatolysis involved observation of the effects of different kinds of injury on motor nerves (Watson, 1974). It was found that changes were more rapid in onset and more marked when the lesion was made closer to the cell body; changes were also more severe when the nerve was cut or ligated, compared with when it was crushed and allowed to reinnervate the distal stump and the target tissue. Suggested causes for these effects include: accumulation of substances normally transported from the cell body; entry of a substance from the circulation at the site of injury; generation of antidromic action potentials at the axotomy site; and interruption of a retrograde trophic effect normally exerted on the neurons by the periphery.

The majority of experiments favour the possibility of a retrograde trophic effect. The evidence is particularly convincing for sympathetic and sensory nerves. It is now apparent that for these nerves the trophic effect is mediated at least in part by Nerve Growth Factor (NGF). Thus in the adult sympathetic ganglion the effects of postganglionic axotomy can be prevented if a pellet releasing NGF is implanted next to the ganglion (Njå & Purves, 1978). More significant is the demonstration that antibodies to NGF produce in the short term some of the changes induced by axotomy, and in the long term (in animals made 'autoimmune' to NGF) the sympathetic neurons atrophy and die (Gorin & Johnson, 1980). Sensory neurons in the same animals do not die but there is a loss of substance P

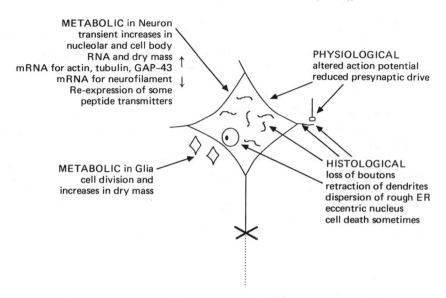

METABOLIC in Neuron
transient increases in
nucleolar and cell body
RNA and dry mass ↑
mRNA for actin, tubulin, GAP-43
mRNA for neurofilament ↓
Re-expression of some
peptide transmitters

PHYSIOLOGICAL
altered action potential
reduced presynaptic drive

METABOLIC in Glia
cell division and
increases in dry mass

HISTOLOGICAL
loss of boutons
retraction of dendrites
dispersion of rough ER
eccentric nucleus
cell death sometimes

Fig. 11.3. Changes in the nerve cell and surrounding glia which are caused directly or indirectly by loss of a retrograde trophic factor following axotomy.

from their central terminals (Schwarz, Pearson & Johnson, 1982), which also occurs after peripheral nerve section (Barbut, Polak & Wall, 1981). Transcription of mRNA for peptide transmitters is much reduced in sensory neurons deprived of NGF (Lindsay & Harman, 1989). Antibodies to NGF also cause the retraction of sensory nerve terminals in the skin of adult rats (Diamond, Holmes & Visheau, 1988). The only possible explanation for these effects is that NGF is essential for sympathetic and sensory function in the adult. Consistent with this explanation is the existence of specific, high-affinity receptors for NGF on the membranes of these neurons, and the fact that NGF taken up by nerve terminals is delivered to the cell body by the fast component of axonal transport (Stockel, Paravicini & Thoenen, 1974). Colchicine applied locally to the axons of a variety of neurons produces the same retrograde changes as axotomy, presumably by interrupting the flow of a retrograde trophic factor (Purves, 1975). Some sympathetically innervated tissues release in culture a substance that is immunologically and biologically indistinguishable from NGF (e.g. Ebendal *et al.*, 1980). Recently it has proved possible to measure low levels of NGF mRNA in tissues innervated by the sympathetic nervous system and to show that blockade of axonal transport leads to a rise in NGF in the tissue and to a fall in the nerve cells innervating it (Heumann, 1987).

Glial cells in culture and degenerating nerve stumps in the animal also release NGF-like material (e.g. Varon, Skaper & Manthorpe, 1981; Lundborg, Longo & Varon, 1982) and 'denervated' Schwann cells develop a rise in the amount of NGF mRNA (Heumann, 1987). This suggests that following injury a retrograde trophic effect might be mediated via NGF released by glial cells surrounding regrowing axons. This may explain why the cell body reaction to injury begins to subside before regenerating sensory axons reach their peripheral targets (Tetzlaff *et al.*, 1988).

Neurons in invertebrates also show changes suggesting that retrograde trophic influences exist. For example, nerve section or interruption of axonal transport with colchicine causes insect motor neuron cell bodies to develop a sodium-sensitive action potential (Pitman, 1975). It has also been shown that individual branches of a single lobster motor neuron have very different presynaptic facilitatory characteristics on the different types of muscle fibre each innervates. This suggests that individual branches of a single neuron can be influenced independently by their muscle fibres (Frank, 1973).

Conclusions

Trophic interactions between neurons and their target cells and glia in the adult nervous system operate continuously to maintain the adult state. The trophic effect of nerve on muscle is mediated predominantly by postsynaptic activity, but the endplate region and other postsynaptic cells are probably maintained by a trophic effect of neurotransmitter or other substances released by nerves. Target and glial cells probably maintain their neurons by means of the same retrograde trophic factors that are molecules required for neuronal survival during development. The evidence for this exists only for sympathetic and sensory neurons but it would seem unlikely that these neurons are unique in a requirement for factors derived from target or glial cells.

Interruption of the trophic interactions produces changes in the properties of the cells. Many of the new properties are reminiscent of the embryonic state: target neurons and muscle become supersensitive to transmitter, glia dedifferentiate and axotomised neurons lose their presynaptic contacts and dendritic complexity. It is therefore likely that the interactions that occur during development to produce maturation of innervation and target cell properties continue to operate in the adult as the trophic interactions maintaining the mature innervated state.

Chapter 12

Nerve growth and synaptic modifications induced by injury

Introduction

Nerve injury in the adult often elicits new nerve outgrowths that can reinnervate and restore function to denervated target tissues. In the peripheral nervous system of nearly all species and the central nervous system of many lower forms, regeneration from the proximal stump usually occurs, and the new outgrowths can be guided back to their original target cells by the structures in the degenerating distal nerve segment. Such regeneration is uncommon in the CNS of mammals, but here and in the peripheral nervous system collateral sprouting from intact axons within a partly denervated target can also develop, and the sprouts emerging at or close to the nerve terminals can reinnervate vacated postsynaptic sites in their near vicinity. Nerve regeneration and nerve sprouting both appear to be controlled predominantly at the site of new growth, probably by factors that stimulate growth and surfaces that guide or permit growth. The nerve cell body also plays a role in regrowth by switching to a metabolic state appropriate for growth.

Nerve injury can also lead to the 'unmasking' of synapses that are functionally ineffective in the normal animal. In some cases tonic activity in a pathway appears to repress the synapses, which are disinhibited as soon as activity is interrupted by injury. In other cases unmasking develops more slowly as cells react to the injury.

Axonal regeneration

Regrowth from the proximal stump of a severed peripheral axon begins within a few hours of injury (Cajal, 1928). In myelinated fibres the growth cones usually emerge from nodes of Ranvier in undamaged parts of the axon just proximal to the lesion. They grow between the Schwann cell basal lamina and the myelin until they reach the lesion site, where many branches may be formed (Friede & Bischhausen, 1980). If the lesion is a nerve crush or freeze, most regenerating axons remain within the Schwann cell basement membrane and collagenous sheath that originally enclosed the intact axon and its Schwann cells (fig. 12.1). Complete reinnervation is therefore usual because the axons are guided back to their original target cells. When

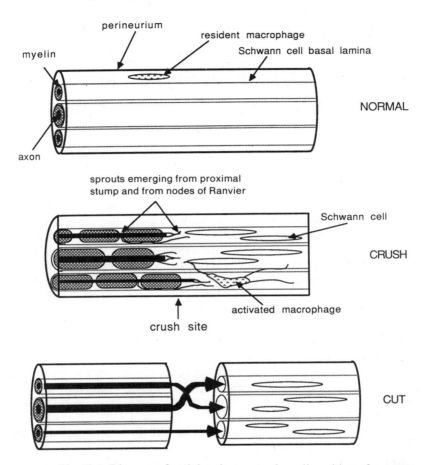

Fig. 12.1. Diagram of peripheral nerve to show disposition of axons, Schwann cells, macrophages, perineurium and Schwann cell sheath in a normal nerve (top), in a crushed nerve (middle) and in a cut nerve (bottom).

a nerve is cut and the cut ends sutured together many axons grow down inappropriate sheaths (fig. 12.1), and restoration of function is therefore poor. In very young mammals, however, there is some evidence that regrowth following motor nerve section must be guided to some extent, for reinnervation is not completely random (Aldskogius & Thomander, 1986; Hardman & Brown, 1987). If the cut ends are not sutured together, glial cells dividing and migrating out from both nerve ends may produce a bridge between the proximal and distal stumps, and axons growing out on these glial cells may still be able to enter the distal stump and hence reach target tissues. In mammals, failure of axons to find the distal stump produces a tangled mass of nervous tissue called a neuroma and a high proportion of sensory neurons in the dorsal root ganglion may die (Aldskogius, Arvidsson & Grant, 1985), but in lower vertebrates axons are capable of continued growth through adjacent tissues and can finally reach and reinnervate their specific targets (Grimm, 1971).

The rate of regrowth in a peripheral nerve is initially slow, but after a few days rates of up to 8 mm per day are possible (Sunderland, 1978). The rate of regrowth is probably determined by the development of an environment conducive to growth in the degenerating stump and by metabolic changes in the cell body.

Among the peripheral features facilitating regrowth are surface bound molecules to which growth cones can adhere; these include laminin in the old Schwann cell basal lamina and N-CAM and L1 (Ng-CAM) (see Chapter 6) on normal unmyelinating Schwann cells (Remak cells) and demyelinated Schwann cells (Daniloff *et al.*, 1986; Martini & Schachner, 1988). Support for regrowth may also come from macrophage-derived Apo-lipoprotein E which may serve as a supplier of lipid (scavenged from degenerating axons) for regenerating axons (Ignatius *et al.*, 1987). Growth factors produced by the denervated, dedifferentiated Schwann cells also appear to be important in regrowth of some types of axon (Varon *et al.*, 1981; Lundborg *et al.*, 1982). NGF in particular is produced by such Schwann cells (Heumann, 1987), and regeneration of peripheral adrenergic axons and axons of the retinal ganglion cells in newts is enhanced by injections of NGF and inhibited by injections of antiserum to NGF (Bjerre, Björklund & Edwards, 1974; Turner & Glaze, 1977; Glaze & Turner, 1978). It has been proposed that NGF is transferred from a low-affinity receptor on the surface of Schwann cells to a high-affinity receptor on the surface of the growth cone (Johnson *et al.*, 1988). The role of growth factors in regeneration of other types of axon is less clear. Regenerating sensory nerves may also need NGF from dedifferentiated Schwann cells, because they grow poorly in a mouse mutant in which the distal nerve stump does not degenerate; regenerating motor axons in the same mutant may not need growth factors because they regrow successfully along the Schwann cells of unmyelinated axons (Brown, Lunn & Perry, 1989, 1990*b*).

The role of the cell body in regeneration has been shown with an experimental paradigm in which growth elicited by a test lesion is compared with that when the nerve has been previously primed with a conditioning lesion made at a more distal site. In peripheral nerves a conditioning lesion produces a significant enhancement of growth of sensory and motor axons (McQuarrie, 1978), indicating that the changes in the cell body following axotomy enhance regeneration. However, regeneration of adrenergic axons is inhibited by a conditioning lesion (McQuarrie *et al.*, 1978). Regeneration of the optic nerve is also enhanced by a conditioning injury, and if the retina is excised and cultured in the presence of NGF the development of axonal outgrowths is markedly advanced and enhanced by a prior lesion to the optic nerve (Turner, Schwab & Thoenen, 1982). It appears, therefore, that the retinal ganglion cell axons develop increased responsiveness to NGF following injury.

Regeneration in the mammalian CNS

Most axons in the CNS regenerate very poorly following injury. The defect seems not to lie in the neurons themselves, for if a segment of peripheral nerve is inserted into the brain, axons of central neurons will invade and grow vigorously along them (Richardson, McGuiness & Aguayo, 1980). The cell body reaction of axotomised neurons in the CNS is also initially identical to that of neurons whose axons project into the periphery but subsequently the rises in actin and tubulin synthesis are markedly depressed (Tetzlaff & Bisby, 1988). Although embryonic monoaminergic and cholinergic neurons transplanted to adult brains can reinnervate and restore function to denervated target neurons (Björklund *et al.*, 1987), they cannot do so unless they are transplanted into or near to the target area. So cells that grow well in culture also find it difficult to make long axonal processes in the adult brain. It seems probable therefore that the environment of the adult mammalian CNS is inimicable to growth for one or more of the following reasons.

> *Lack of endoneurial sheaths.* These exist only in the periphery, where they guide regenerating axons very successfully.
> *Lack of growth stimuli.* The oligodendroglia (the CNS equivalent of Schwann cells) may fail to provide either the surface attached molecules needed for growth cone attachment or the soluble molecules needed to maintain the cell body during regrowth and to attract the growth cones.
> *Production of growth inhibitors.* Factors or surfaces directly inhibitory to growth may be produced by astrocytes (Smith, Miller & Silver, 1986) or oligodendroglia and CNS myelin (Schwab & Caroni, 1988; Fawcett, Rokos & Bakst, 1989). These could act by suppressing the cell body reaction or inhibiting growth cone attachment. Evidence for this is the observation that antibodies against a myelin-associated inhibitory protein can allow some degree of long axon regrowth (Caroni & Schwab, 1988).
> *Formation of scar tissue* at the site of injury may contribute to poor central regeneration. This is suggested by the successful regeneration of central monoaminergic axons following chemical axotomy with 6–hydroxydopamine, which leaves surrounding tissues intact (Nobin *et al.*, 1973).

Collateral sprouting

Intact axons, not directly involved in damage, can respond to the denervation of neighbouring territory by developing new outgrowths (collateral sprouts) that innervate the denervated neurons or tissue. This was first suspected at the turn of the century when it was found that partly denervated muscles recovered their strength quickly and contained few atrophied muscle fibres, even before the cut axons had regenerated. In the 1950s, histological investigations of partly denervated muscles (Hoffmann, 1950) and ganglia stained with silver confirmed that the denervated target cells had become reinnervated by outgrowths from the remaining intact axons. Similar recovery following partial denervation in the peripheral nervous system has been demonstrated in some skin sensory nerves (e.g. Devor *et al.*, 1979) and in autonomic ganglia (Murray & Thompson, 1957; Courtney & Roper, 1976).

The first attempts to detect sprouting in the CNS were made in the spinal cord after section of some of the dorsal roots, but these studies produced equivocal results because of limitations in the techniques used (Liu & Chambers, 1958; Goldberger & Murray, 1982). However, more recent studies have confirmed the presence of expanded field territories of intact dorsal root ganglion cells in the spinal cord following pronase-induced dorsal root ganglion cell death (LaMotte, Kopodia & Kocol, 1989) and it is now clear that injury-induced sprouting also occurs at many other CNS loci (see Björklund & Stenevi, 1979). The direct histological methods used to detect the sprouting include axon stains, axon tracers, stains specific for transmitter and transmitter enzymes, and electron microscopy to visualise synapses produced by the sprouts (e.g. Raisman & Field, 1973). Electrophysiological recording has shown that at least some of these synapses can transmit (e.g. Lynch, Deadwyler & Cotman, 1973), and in several studies behavioural assay has revealed that the loss of function produced by a nerve lesion is partly restored following sprouting (e.g. Goldberger, 1977; Loesche & Steward, 1977). Sprouting may therefore help to account for some of the recovery following brain damage, but it might also contribute to less beneficial effects, such as spasticity.

Sprouting in the CNS of developing animals is vigorous and the sprouts can travel long distances (e.g. Tsukahara, 1981). Sprouting in the CNS of adults is in contrast much less pronounced: many nerves do not sprout and the sprouts of those that do probably remain localised to the dendrites that have been deafferented (Cotman, Nieto Sampedro & Harris, 1981). Presumably the same factors that limit regeneration in the CNS also limit sprouting.

Investigation of the process of sprouting has been made predominantly on motor neurons, cutaneous afferents and preganglionic sympathetic fibres, whose peripheral location makes experimentation easier. In partly denervated muscles it is possible to distinguish new outgrowths arising either from nodes of Ranvier, (*nodal sprouts*) or from the nerve terminals themselves (*terminal sprouts*) (Hoffman, 1950), (fig. 12.2). In most muscles nodal sprouts predominate; these cross into the endoneurial sheaths, vacated as the result of partial denervation, and grow distally towards denervated endplates. Sprouting begins two to three days after partial denervation and may be complete in several weeks in small animals.

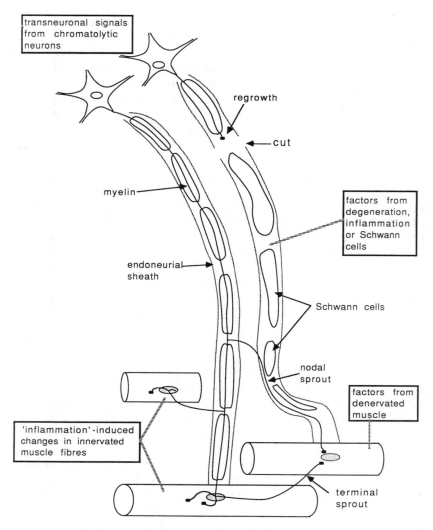

Fig. 12.2. Collateral sprouting following partial denervation. Factors likely to be involved in causing sprouting are shown in the boxes.

Surprisingly, there appears to be no cell body reaction associated with sprouting (Pamphlett, 1988). There also appears to be a limit to the number of extra synapses that a motor neuron can establish or maintain with sprouts and many are eliminated if the original axons regenerate to the endplates (Brown & Ironton, 1978). Similar observations have been made on sprouting of preganglionic axons in the superior cervical ganglion (Leistol *et al.*, 1986). In partly denervated skin only the nociceptive afferents sprout (Jackson & Diamond, 1983; Kinnamon & Aldskogius, 1986); the sprouting is accelerated by electrical activity and inhibited by blockade of activity (Doucette & Diamond, 1987).

Several changes in the partly denervated tissue and in the pool of neurons innervating it could be responsible for the initiation of collateral sprouting (fig. 12.2). It was thought originally that sprouting might be stimulated by the release of some breakdown product of degenerating axons or myelin. However, sprouting is observed without degeneration when muscles are rendered inactive by various means (Duchen & Strich, 1968; Brown & Ironton, 1977; Hopkins, Brown & Keynes, 1981), implying that muscle fibres produce the stimulus. This is reinforced by the finding that selective destruction of muscle fibres at the time of partial denervation inhibits subsequent nodal sprouting (Keynes, Hopkins & Brown, 1983). An appealing idea is that the stimulus for sprouting is the same target-derived growth factor thought to be responsible for survival of neurons and axon branches during development. The recent observation that sprouting of cutaneous nociceptive afferents is inhibited by antibodies to NGF is consistent with this view (Diamond *et al.*, 1987). For motor neurons the equivalent factor is unknown, but it might be an insulin-like growth factor (IGF-II), mRNA for which is expressed in foetal and denervated muscles (Ishii, 1989).

The stimulus for terminal sprouting in muscle appears to have a very limited range of diffusion (Brown *et al.*, 1980; Slack & Pockett, 1981). This could be explained if terminal sprouting requires the presence of a molecule that is released by inactive or denervated fibres, that binds tightly to the surface of muscle fibres, and that stimulates growth by providing a suitable substrate for attachment of sprouts. A promising candidate is N-CAM, a molecule that can act as a substrate for growth cones (Chapter 5): this appears in inactive muscles, and antibodies to it can partly suppress terminal sprout growth (Booth, Kemplay & Brown, 1990). Nodal sprouts may have a similar need for a suitable growth surface, provided in partly denervated muscles by the 'denervated' Schwann cells.

In mammalian muscles examined so far, the strict localisation of sprouting to the vicinity of denervated fibres within a partly denervated muscle rules out any significant effect of a sprouting stimulus passing from axotomised to intact motor neurons in the spinal cord. However, in frogs denervation of one muscle can cause sprouting or changes in synaptic effectiveness in muscles on the other side of the animal, so it appears that some signal for growth can spread across the spinal cord (Rotshenker, 1979; Herrera & Grinnell, 1981; Herrera, Grinnell & Wolowske, 1985; Herrera & Scott, 1985).

Unmasking of suppressed synapses

The novel concept of structurally normal but functionally inactive synapses was first raised to prominence following experiments on the reinnervation of denervated eye muscles in fish (Mark, 1970). The results of these experiments suggested that the terminals of a foreign nerve that had innervated the muscles were not withdrawn when the correct nerve regenerated; instead it appeared that they remained on the fibres as 'silent' synapses that could be quickly reactivated or 'unmasked' if the correct nerve was cut a second time. Although more careful investigation showed that functionally suppressed synapses were not present in either the fish eye muscles (Scott, 1975) or in comparable reinnervated amphibian muscles (Dennis & Yip, 1978), there is nevertheless now considerable evidence for the existence of such synapses in the CNS.

Examples of rapidly induced changes in the visual system that can be attributed to de-repression of suppressed synapses in the visual cortex have been discussed already in Chapter 9 and there are also numerous examples from elsewhere in the CNS. Cells in the dorsal column nuclei (a sensory relay in the spinal cord) develop novel receptive fields immediately if their normal inputs are cut in the dorsal roots or blocked by local cooling in the cord (Dostrovsky, Millar & Wall, 1976). The fact that these changes occur so quickly implies that the new receptive fields arise from pre-existing ineffective synapses which become effective when tonic activity in the other sensory axons is interrupted. Subliminal inputs can also be revealed by electrical stimulation of sensory nerves (Dostrovsky, Jabbur & Millar, 1978) and immediate changes in receptive fields occur if the level of excitability of cells and presynaptic terminals in the dorsal column is increased by infusion of 4–aminopyridine (Saade *et al.*, 1982). The presence of normally ineffective sensory synapses in the spinal cord of the rat has been confirmed by raising general levels of neuronal excitability by pharmacological means or by using repetitive electrical stimulation (Markus & Pomeranz, 1987).

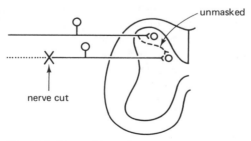

Fig. 12.3. Unmasking of silent synapses on dorsal horn neurons following section of a peripheral nerve.

Section of a peripheral sensory nerve in rats also produces within a week new receptive fields on dorsal horn cells that are normally driven only by the sectioned nerve (Devor & Wall, 1981; fig. 12.3). The evidence favours unmasking of previously ineffective synapses, because sprouting of the intact afferents could not be detected in the cord with a stain specific for some sensory nerve terminals (Devor & Claman, 1980) or by following the spinal distribution of neighbouring intact nerves after trans-ganglionic transport of HRP (Selzer & Devor, 1984). An early decrease in the dorsal root potential in the roots of the damaged nerve paralleled the development of the new receptive fields, so it is likely that decreased 'surround' presynaptic inhibition is responsible for unmasking the synapses (Wall & Devor, 1981). Substance P could be the neurotransmitter mediating surround inhibition, because there is an early loss of substance P from sensory terminals following a cut injury (Barbut *et al.*, 1981). The signal for unmasking may be associated with the uptake by the nerve of some substance from the circulation, because the new receptive fields do not develop if the peripheral nerve is crushed rather than cut (Devor & Wall, 1981). It is more likely, however, that unmasking is associated with the metabolic and structural changes in the dorsal root ganglion cells that accompany interruption of a retrograde trophic factor, probably Nerve Growth Factor. After a crush lesion the axons gain very rapid access to a large source of Nerve Growth Factor in the distal nerve stump (Heumann, 1987) which is not available after a cut. Other studies in which extensive peripheral denervation was used have failed to uncover any plasticity amongst connections from skin afferents to dorsal horn neurons projecting in the spinocervical tract (A.G.Brown *et al.*, 1984). This may reflect the limited extent of incoming axonal arbours. Small peripheral denervations are followed after some weeks by reorganisation of receptive fields in the cat dorsal horn (Wilson & Snow, 1987) but this may be due to axonal sprouting rather than reactivation of previously silent synapses.

Immediate changes in receptive fields of cortical neurons have been observed in the cat after applying an epidural block to lumbar nerve roots (Metzler & Marks, 1979). Section of peripheral nerves also produces an immediate change in cortical receptive fields of remaining nerves in monkeys and there is an additional slower and orderly expansion of their somatotopic projection which has been attributed to de-repression of pre-existing synapses rather than frank sprouting (Merzenich *et al.*, 1988). The evidence is the following: thalamic afferent terminal arbours are wider than physiologically recorded receptive field sizes; block of inhibitory transmission can produce very large receptive fields; intracellular recording from cortical cells reveals that excitatory postsynaptic potentials can be evoked from wider areas of skin than can evoke action potentials; finally, continuous electrical stimulation of one peripheral nerve can, over the course of minutes to hours, result in a very large increase in the size of receptive fields.

The mechanisms of synaptic repression and unmasking are still matters for conjecture. Mutual repression of synaptic transmission has been observed on multiply-innervated muscle fibres (e.g. Trussell & Grinnell, 1985), and a similar phenomenon could occur on central neurons. Various kinds of synaptic inhibitory circuits could contribute to repression and unmasking of inputs. Electrical activity must also be involved where the disinhibition is immediate and longer-term unmasking might also be produced by modifications of synaptic efficacy by patterns of activity. Changes in trophic support might also contribute to the longer term changes in connections. The significance of suppressed synapses is also unclear. They may help maintain sensation following peripheral nerve injury and at higher levels in the brain they may play a part in adaptations to changing sensory environments and possibly in learning and memory.

References

Abrams, T.W. & Kandel, E.R. (1988). Is contiguity detection in classical conditioning a system or a cellular property? Learning in *Aplysia* suggests a possible molecular site. *Trends in Neurosciences*, **11**, 128–35.

Acheson, A. & Rutishauser, U. (1988). Neural cell adhesion molecule regulates cell contact-mediated changes on choline acetyltransferase activity of embryonic chick sympathetic neurons. *Journal of Cell Biology*, **106**, 479–86.

Adler, R., Manthorpe, M., Skaper, S.D. & Varon, S. (1981). Polyornithine attached neurite promoting factors (PNPFS). Culture sources and responsive neurons. *Brain Research*, **206**, 129–44.

Akam, M. (1987). The molecular basis for metameric pattern in the *Drosophila* embryo. *Development*, **101**, 1–22.

Alberts, B., Bray, D., Lewis, J., Raff, M., Roberts, K. & Watson, J.D. (1989). *Molecular Biology of the Cell*. 2nd edition. New York and London, Garland.

Albuquerque, E.X., Schuh, F.T. & Kauffman, F.C. (1971). Early membrane depolarisation of the fast mammalian muscle after denervation. *Pflugers Archiv. European Journal of Physiology*, **328**, 36–50.

Albus, J.S. (1971). A theory of cerebellar function. *Mathematical Biosciences*, **10**, 25–61.

Aldskogius, H., Arvidsson, J. & Grant, G. (1985). The reaction of primary sensory neurons to peripheral nerve injury with particular emphasis on transganglionic changes. *Brain Research Review*, **10**, 27–46.

Aldskogius, H. & Thomander, L. (1986). Selective reinnervation of somatotopically appropriate muscles after facial nerve transection and regeneration in neonatal rats. *Brain Research*, **375**, 126–34.

Altman, J. (1972). Postnatal development of the cerebellar cortex of the rat. *Journal of Comparative Neurology*, **145**, 353–98.

Andersen, P. (1982). Cerebellar synaptic plasticity. *Trends in Neurosciences*, **5**, 324–5.

Andersen, P., Blackstad, T., Hulleberg, G., Trommald, M. & Vaaland, J.L. (1987). Dimensions of dendritic spines of rat dentate granule cells during long-term potentiation. *Journal of Physiology*, **390**, 264P.

Anderson, D.J. (1989). The neural crest cell lineage problem: neuropoiesis? *Neuron*, **3**, 1–12.

Anderson, H., Edwards, J.S. & Palka, J. (1980). Developmental neurobiology of invertebrates. *Annual Review of Neuroscience*, **3**, 97–139.

Anderson, M.J. & Cohen, M.W. (1977). Nerve induced and spontaneous redistribution of acetylcholine receptors on cultured muscle cells. *Journal of Physiology*, **268**, 757–73.

139

Angevine, J.B. & Sidman, B.L. (1961). Autoradiographic study of cell migration during histogenesis of cerebral cortex in the mouse. *Nature*, **192**, 766–8.

Antonicek, H., Persohn, E. & Schachner, M. (1987). Biochemical and functional characterisation of a novel neuron–glia adhesion molecule that is involved in neuronal migration. *Journal of Cell Biology*, **104**, 1587–95.

Anwyl, R. (1989). Protein kinase C and long-term potentiation. *Trends in Pharmacological Sciences*, **10**, 236–8.

Ashkenazi, A., Ramachandran, J. & Capon, D.J. (1989). Acetylcholine analogue stimulates DNA synthesis in brain-derived cells via specific muscarinic subtypes. *Nature*, **340**, 146–50.

Bagust, J., Lewis, D.M. & Westerman, R.A. (1973). Polyneuronal innervation of kitten skeletal muscle. *Journal of Physiology*, **229**, 241–55.

Bailey, C.H. & Chen, M. (1989). Time course of structural changes at identified sensory neuron synapses during long-term sensitization in *Aplysia*. *Journal of Neuroscience*, **9**, 1774–80.

Bailey, C.H., Hawkins, R.D., Chen, M.C. & Kandel, E.R. (1981). Interneurons involved in mediation and modulation of gill-withdrawal reflex in *Aplysia*. IV. Morphological basis of pre-synaptic facilitation. *Journal of Neurophysiology*, **45**, 340–60.

Bamburg, J.R., Bray, D. & Chapman, K. (1986). Assembly of microtubules at the tip of growing axons. *Nature*, **321**, 788–90.

Banker, G.A. & Cowan, W.M. (1979). Further observations on hippocampal neurons in dispersed cell culture. *Journal of Comparative Neurology*, **187**, 469–94.

Banks, M.S., Aslin, R.N. & Letson, R.D. (1975). Sensitive period for the development of human binocular vision. *Science*, **190**, 675–7.

Barbera, A.J., Marchase, R.B. & Roth, S. (1973). Adhesive recognition and retinotectal specificity. *Proceedings of the National Academy of Science U.S.A.*, **70**, 2482–6.

Barbin, G., Manthorpe, M. & Varon, S. (1984). Purification of the chick eye ciliary neuronotrophic factor. *Journal of Neurochemistry*, **43**, 1468–78.

Barbut, D., Polak, J. & Wall, P.D. (1981). Substance P in spinal cord dorsal horn decreases following peripheral nerve injury. *Brain Research*, **205**, 289–98.

Barde, Y.A. (1988). What, if anything, is a neurotrophic factor? *Trends in Neurosciences*, **11**, 343–6.

(1989). Trophic factors and neuronal survival. *Neuron*, **2**, 1525–34.

Barnes, D.M. (1988). Cells without growth factors commit suicide. *Science*, **242**, 1510–11.

Baroffio, A., Dupin, E. & Le Douarin, N.M. (1988). Clone-forming ability and differentiation potential of migratory neural crest cells. *Proceedings of the National Academy of Science U.S.A.*, **85**, 5325–9.

Barzilai, A., Kennedy, T.E., Sweatt, J.D. & Kandel, E.R. (1989). 5–HT modulates protein synthesis and the expression of specific proteins during long-term facilitation in aplysia sensory neurons. *Neuron*, **2**, 1577–86.

Bastiani, M.J., Doe, C.Q., Helfand, S.L. & Goodman, C.S. (1985). Neuronal specificity and growth cone guidance in grasshopper. *Trends in Neurosciences*, **8**, 257–66.

Bastiani, M.J., Harrelson, A.L., Snow, P.M. & Goodman, C.S. (1987). Expression of fasciclin I and II glycoproteins on subsets of axon pathways during neuronal development in the grasshopper. *Cell*, **48**, 745–75.

Bate, C.M. (1976). Pioneer neurons in an insect embryo. *Nature*, **260**, 54–6.

Bear, M.F. & Singer, W. (1986). Modulation of visual cortical plasticity by acetylcholine and noradrenaline. *Nature*, **320**, 172–6.

Bennett, M.R., Lai, K. & Nurcombe, V. (1980). Identification of embryonic motor neurons in vitro: their survival is dependent on skeletal muscle. *Brain Research*, **190**, 537–42.

Bennett, M.R. & Lavidis, N.A. (1982). Development of the topographical projection of motor neurons to amphibian muscle accompanies motor neuron death. *Developmental Brain Research*, **2**, 448–52.

   (1984). Development of the topographical projection of motor neurons to a rat muscle accompanies loss of polyneuronal innervation. *Journal of Neuroscience*, **4**, 2204–12.

Bennett, M.R. & Lavidis, N. (1986). Topographical projections of segmental nerves to the frog gluteus muscle during loss of polyneuronal innervation. *Journal of Physiology*, **375**, 303–26.

Bennett, M.R., McClachlan, E.M. & Taylor, R.S. (1973). The formation of synapses in reinnervated mammalian striated muscle. *Journal of Physiology*, **233**, 481–500.

Bennett, M.R. & Robinson, J. (1989). Growth and elimination of nerve terminals at synaptic sites during polyneuronal innervation of muscle cells: a trophic hypothesis. *Proceedings of the Royal Society of London*, **B235**, 299–320.

Benoit, P. & Changeux, J. P. (1975). Consequences of tenotomy on the evolution of multi innervation in developing rat soleus muscle. *Brain Research*, **99**, 345–58.

Beresford, B. (1983). Brachial muscles in the chick embryo: the fate of individual somites. *Journal of Embryology and Experimental Morphology*, **77**, 99–116.

Berlot, J. & Goodman, C.S. (1984). Guidance of peripheral pioneer neurons in the grasshopper. *Science*, **223**, 493–6.

Bernhardt, R. & Easter, S.S. (1988). Regenerated optic fibres in goldfish reestablish a crude sectoral order in the visual pathway. *Journal of Comparative Neurology*, **277**, 403–19.

Betz, W.J., Caldwell, J.H. & Ribchester, R.R. (1980). The effects of partial denervation at birth on the development of muscle fibres and motor units in rat lumbrical muscle. *Journal of Physiology*, **303**, 265–80.

Beuche, W. & Friede, R.L. (1984). The role of non-resident cells in Wallerian degeneration. *Journal of Neurocytology*, **13**, 767–96.

Bixby, J.L. (1981). Ultrastructural observations on synapse elimination in neonatal rabbit skeletal muscle. *Journal of Neurocytology*, **10**, 81–100.

Bixby, J.L., Pratt, R.S., Lilien, J. & Reichardt, L.F. (1987). Neurite outgrowth on muscle cell surfaces involves matrix receptors as well as Ca^{2+}-dependent and -independent cell adhesion molecules. *Proceedings of the National Academy of Science U.S.A.*, **84**, 2555–9.

Bixby, J.L. & Van Essen, D.C. (1979). Competition between foreign and original nerves in adult mammalian skeletal muscle. *Nature*, **282**, 726–8.

Bjerre, B., Björklund, A. & Edwards, D.C. (1974). Axonal regeneration of peripheral adrenergic neurons; effects of antiserum to NGF in mouse. *Cell and Tissue Research*, **148**, 441–76.

Björklund, A. & Stenevi, U. (1979). Regeneration of monoaminergic and cholinergic neurons in the mammalian central nervous system. *Physiological Reviews*, **59**, 62–97.

Björklund, A., Lundvall, O., Isacson, O., Brundin, P., Wictorin, K., Strecker, R.E.,

Clarke, D.J. & Dunnett, S.B. (1987). Mechanisms of action of intracerebral neural implants: studies on nigral and striatal grafts to the lesioned striatum. *Trends in Neurosciences*, **10**, 509–16.

Black, I.B., Chikaraishi, D.M. & Lewis, E.J. (1985). Trans-synaptic increase in RNA coding for tyrosine hydroxylase in a rat sympathetic ganglion. *Brain Research*, **339**, 151–3.

Black, M.M. & Baas, P.W. (1989). The basis of polarity in neurons. *Trends in Neurosciences*, **12**, 211–14.

Blair, S. & Palka, J. (1985). Axon guidance in the wing of *Drosophila*. *Trends in Neurosciences*, **8**, 284–8.

Blakemore, C. & Cooper, G.F. (1970). Development of the brain depends on the visual environment. *Nature*, **228**, 477–8.

Blakemore, C. & Mitchell, D.E. (1973). Environmental modification of the visual cortex and the neural basis of learning and memory. *Nature*, **241**, 467–8.

Blakemore, C. & Vital Durand, F. (1983). Visual deprivation prevents the postnatal maturation of spatial resolution and contrast sensitivity for neurons of the monkey's striate cortex. *Journal of Physiology*, **345**, 40P.

(1986). Effects of visual deprivation on the development of the monkey's lateral geniculate nucleus. *Journal of Physiology*, **380**, 493–511.

Bliss, R.V.P. & Lømo, T. (1973). Long-lasting potentiation of synaptic transmission in the dentate area of the anaesthetised rabbit following stimulation of the perforant path. *Journal of Physiology*, **232**, 331–6.

Booth, C.M. & Brown, M.C. (1988). Localization of neural cell adhesion molecule in denervated muscle to both the plasma membrane and extracellular compartments by immuno-electron microscopy. *Neuroscience*, **27**, 699–709.

Booth, C.M., Kemplay, S. & Brown, M.C. (1990). An antibody to neural cell adhesion molecule impairs motor nerve terminal sprouting in a mouse muscle locally paralysed with botulinum toxin. *Neuroscience*, **35**, 85–91.

Borasio, G.D., John, J., Wittinghofer, A., Barde, Y.A., Sendtner, M. & Heumann, R. (1989). ras p21 protein promotes survival and fiber outgrowth of cultured embryonic neurons. *Neuron*, **2**, 1087–96.

Bostock, H. & Sears, T.A. (1978). The internodal axon membrane: electrical excitability and continuous conduction in segmental demyelination. *Journal of Physiology*, **280**, 273–301.

Bray, D. (1973). Model for membrane movements in the neural growth cone. *Nature*, **244**, 93–5.

Bray, G.M., Rasminsky, M. & Aguayo, A.J. (1981). Interaction between axons and their sheath cells. *Annual Review of Neuroscience*, **4**, 127–62.

Breedlove, S.M. & Arnold, A.P. (1983a). Hormonal control of a developing neuromuscular system. I.Complete demasculinization of the male rat spinal nucleus of bulbocavernosus using the anti-androgen flutamide. *Journal of Neuroscience*, **3**, 417–23.

(1983b). Hormonal control of a developing neuromuscular system. II.Sensitive periods for the androgen-induced masculinization of the rat spinal nucleus of the bulbocavernosus. *Journal of Neuroscience*, **3**, 424–32.

Brenner, H.R., Meier, T. & Widmer, B. (1983). Early action of nerve determines motor endplate differentiation in rat muscle. *Nature*, **305**, 536–7.

Brockes, J.P. (1984). Mitogenic growth factors and nerve dependence of limb regeneration. *Science*, **225**, 1280–6.

Brockes, J.P. & Kintner, C.R. (1986). Glial growth factor and nerve-dependent proliferation in the regeneration blastema of urodele amphibians. *Cell*, **45**, 301–6.

Brockes, J.P. & Lemke, G.E. (1981). The neuron as a source of mitogen: its influence on the proliferation of glial and non-neural cells. In *Development in the Nervous System*, (ed. D.R.Garrod & J.D.Feldman), pp. 309–27. Cambridge, Cambridge University Press.

Bronner-Fraser, M. (1986). An antibody to a receptor for fibronectin and laminin perturbs cranial neural crest development in vivo. *Developmental Biology*, **117**, 528–36.

(1987). Perturbation of cranial neural crest migration by the HNK-1 antibody. *Developmental Biology*, **123**, 321–31.

(1988). A monoclonal antibody against a laminin–heparan sulfate proteoglycan complex perturbs cranial neural crest migration in vivo. *Journal of Cell Biology*, **106**, 1321–9.

Bronner-Fraser, M. & Fraser, S.E. (1988). Cell lineage analysis reveals multipotency of some avian neural crest cells. *Nature*, **335**, 161–4.

Brown, A.G., Fyffe, R.E.W., Noble, R. & Rowe, M.J. (1984). Effects of hindlimb nerve sections on lumbosacral dorsal horn neurones in the cat. *Journal of Physiology*, **354**, 375–94.

Brown, M.C. & Booth, C.M. (1983). Postnatal development of the adult pattern of motor axon distribution in rat muscle. *Nature*, **304**, 741–2.

Brown, M.C., Holland, R.L. & Hopkins, W.G. (1981). Restoration of focal multiple innervation in rat muscles by transmission block during a critical stage of development. *Journal of Physiology*, **318**, 355–64.

Brown, M.C., Holland, R.L., Hopkins, W.G. & Keynes, R.J. (1980). An assessment of the spread of the signal for terminal sprouting within and between muscles. *Brain Research*, **210**, 145–51.

Brown, M.C., Hopkins, W.G. & Keynes, R.J. (1982a). Importance of pathway formation for nodal sprout production in partly denervated muscles. *Brain Research*, **243**, 345–9.

(1982b). Comparison of the effects of denervation and botulinum toxin paralysis on muscle properties in mice. *Journal of Physiology*, **327**, 29–37.

Brown, M.C. & Ironton, R. (1977). Motor neurone sprouting induced by prolonged tetrodotoxin block of nerve action potentials. *Nature*, **265**, 459–61.

(1978). Sprouting and regression of neuromuscular synapses in partially denervated mammalian muscles. *Journal of Physiology*, **278**, 325–8.

Brown, M.C., Jansen, J.K.S. & Van Essen, D. (1976). Polyneuronal innervation of skeletal muscle in new born rats and its elimination during maturation. *Journal of Physiology*, **261**, 387–442.

Brown, M.C., Lunn, E.R. & Perry, V.H. (1989). The route taken by motor axons growing down an intact distal nerve stump in mice. *Journal of Physiology*, **418**, 148P.

(1990). Failure of normal Wallerian degeneration results in very poor regeneration of cutaneous afferent fibres in mice. *Journal of Physiology*, **422**, 12P.

Brown, T.H., Chapman, P.F., Kairiss, E.W. & Keenan, C.L. (1988). Long-term synaptic potentiation. *Science*, **242**, 724–8.

Brunelli, M., Castellucci, V. & Kandel, E.R. (1976). Synaptic facilitation and behavioural sensitization in *Aplysia*: possible role of serotonin and cyclic AMP. *Science*, **194**, 1178–81.

Buller, A.J., Eccles, J.C. & Eccles, R.M. (1960). Interaction between motor neurones and muscles in respect of the characteristic speeds of their responses. *Journal of Physiology*, **150**, 417–39.

Bunge, M.B., Wood, P.M., Tynan, L.B., Bates, M.L. & Sanes, J.R. (1989). Perineurium originates from fibroblasts: demonstration in vitro with a retroviral marker. *Science*, **243**, 229–31.

Bunt, S.M. & Lund, R.D. (1981). Development of a transient retino retinal pathway in hooded and albino rats. *Brain Research*, **211**, 399–404.

Burden, S.J., Sargent, P.B. & McMahan, U.J. (1979). Acetylcholine receptors in regenerating muscle accumulate at original synaptic sites in the absence of the nerve. *Journal of Cell Biology*, **82**, 412–25.

Burke, R.E. (1981). Motor Units: anatomy, physiology and functional organisation. In *Handbook of Physiology*, Section 1, Volume II, pp. 345–422. Bethesda, American Physiological Society.

Burnstock, G. (1981). Neurotransmitters and trophic factors in the autonomic nervous system. *Journal of Physiology*, **313**, 1–35.

Cabrera, C.V., Martinez Arias, A. & Bate, M. (1987). The expression of three members of the achaete–scute gene complex correlates with neuroblast segregation in *Drosophila*. *Cell*, **50**, 425–33.

Cajal, S.R.y. (1928). *Degeneration and regeneration of the nervous system*. Translated by R.M. May. London, Oxford University Press.

Callaway, E.M., Soha, J.M. & Van Essen, D.C. (1987). Competition favouring inactive over active motor neurons during synapse elimination. *Nature*, **328**, 422–6.

Callaway, E.M. & Van Essen, D.C. (1989). Slowing of synapse elimination by α-bungarotoxin superfusion of the neonatal rabbit soleus muscle. *Developmental Biology*, **131**, 356–65.

Campenot, R.B. (1977). Local control of neurite development by nerve growth factor. *Proceedings of the National Academy of Science U.S.A.*, **74**, 4516–9.

(1985). The regulation of nerve fibre length by intercalated elongation and retraction. *Developmental Brain Research*, **20**, 149–84.

Campos Ortega, J.A. (1988). Cellular interactions during early neurogenesis of *Drosophila melanogaster*. *Trends in Neurosciences*, **11**, 400–5.

Cangiano, A. (1985). Denervation supersensitivity as a model for the neural control of muscle. *Neurosciences*, **14**, 963–71.

Cangiano, A. & Lutzemberger, L. (1980). Partial denervation in inactive muscle affects innervated and denervated fibres equally. *Nature*, **285**, 233–5.

Carbonetto, S., Evans, D. & Cochard, P. (1987). Nerve fiber growth in culture on tissue substrates from central and peripheral nervous system. *Journal of Neuroscience*, **7**, 610–20.

Carew, T.J., Walters, E.T. & Kandel, E.R. (1981). Classical conditioning in a simple withdrawal reflex in *Aplysia californica*. *Journal of Neuroscience*, **1**, 1426–37.

Caroni, P. & Schwab, M.E. (1988). Antibody against myelin-associated inhibitor of neurite growth neutralizes non-permissive substrate properties of CNS white matter. *Neuron*, **1**, 85–96.

Castellucci, V. & Kandel, E.R. (1976). Pre-synaptic facilitation as a mechanism for behavioural sensitization in *Aplysia*. *Science*, **194**, 1176–8.

Caviness, V.S. (1982). Neocortical histogenesis in normal and reeler mice: a developmental study based upon ^{3}H-thymidine autoradiography. *Developmental Brain Research*, **4**, 293–302.

Chalazonitis, A. & Zigmond, R.E. (1980). Effects of synaptic and antidromic stimulation on tyrosine hydroxylase activity in the rat superior cervical ganglion. *Journal of Physiology*, **300**, 525–38.

Chang, S., Rathjen, F.G. & Raper, J.A. (1987). Extension of neurites on axons is impaired by antibodies against specific nerve cell surface glycoproteins. *Journal of Cell Biology*, **104**, 355–62.

Chevalier, A., Kieny, M. & Mauger, A. (1977). Limb–somite relationship: origin of the limb musculature. *Journal of Embryology and Experimental Morphology*, **41**, 245–58.

Chiu, A.Y., Matthew, W.D. & Patterson, P.H. (1986). A monoclonal antibody that blocks the activity of a neurite regeneration-promoting factor: studies on the binding site and its localization in vivo. *Journal of Cell Biology*, **163**, 1383–98.

Chiu, A.Y. & Sanes, J.R. (1984). Development of basal lamina in synaptic and extra synaptic portions of embryonic rat muscle. *Developmental Biology*, **103**, 456–67.

Chow, I. & Poo, M.N. (1985). Release of acetylcholine from embryonic neurons upon contact with muscle cell. *Journal of Neuroscience*, **5**, 1076–82.

Chun, J.J.M., Nakamura, M.J. & Shatz, C.J. (1987). Transient cells of the developing mammalian telencephalon are peptide-immunoreactive neurons. *Nature*, **325**, 617–9.

Chuong, C.M., Crossin, K.L. & Edelman, G.M. (1987). Sequential expression and differential function of multiple adhesion molecules during the formation of cerebellar cortical layers. *Journal of Cell Biology*, **104**, 331–42.

Clarke, P.G.H. (1981). Chance, repetition and error in the development of the nervous system. *Perspectives in Biology and Medicine*, **25**, 2–19.

Clarke, P.G.H. & Cowan, W.M. (1976). The development of the isthmo optic tract in the chick, with special reference to the occurrence and correction of developmental errors in the location and connections of isthmo optic neurons. *Journal of Comparative Neurology*, **167**, 143–64.

Cohen, J., Nurcombe, V., Jeffrey, P. & Edgar, D. (1989). Developmental loss of functional laminin receptors on retinal ganglion cells is regulated by their target tissues. *Development*, **107**, 381–7.

Cohen, M.W. (1972). The development of neurotransmitter connections in the presence of d-tubocurarine. *Brain Research*, **41**, 457–63.

Cohen, M.W. & Weldon, P.R. (1980). Localization of acetylcholine receptors and synaptic ultrastructure at nerve muscle contacts in culture: Dependence on nerve type. *Journal of Cell Biology*, **86**, 388–401.

Cole, G.J. & Glaser, L. (1986). A heparin-binding domain from N-CAM is involved in neural cell–substratum adhesion. *Journal of Cell Biology*, **102**, 403–12.

Collingridge, G. (1987). The role of NMDA receptors in learning and memory. *Nature*, **330**, 604–5.

Collingridge, G.L. & Bliss, T.V.P. (1987). NMDA receptors – their role in long-term potentiation. *Trends in Neurosciences*, **10**, 228–9.

Cooper, K.E., Ferguson, A.V. & Veale, W.L. (1980). Modification of thermoregulatory responses in rabbits reared at elevated environmental temperatures. *Journal of Physiology*, **303**, 165–72.

Cornbrooks, C.J., Carey, D.L., McDonald, J.A., Timpl, R. & Bunge, R.P. (1983). In vivo and in vitro observations on laminin production by Schwann cells. *Proceedings of the National Academy of Science U.S.A.*, **80**, 3850–4.

Cotman, C.W., Nieto Sampedro, M. & Harris, E.W. (1981). Synapse replacement in the nervous system of adult vertebrates. *Physiological Reviews*, **61**, 684–784.

Courtney, K. & Roper, S. (1976). Sprouting of synapses after partial denervation of frog cardiac ganglion. *Nature*, **259**, 317–9.

Covault, J. & Sanes, J.R. (1985). Neural cell adhesion molecule (N-CAM) accumulates in denervated and paralyzed skeletal muscles. *Proceedings of the National Academy of Science U.S.A.*, **82**, 4544–5548.

Cowan, W.M. (1973). Neuronal death as a regulative mechanism in the control of cell number in the nervous system. In *Development and Aging in the Nervous System* (ed. M. Rockstein), pp. 19–41. New York, Academic Press.

Crang, A.J. & Blakemore, W.F. (1986). Observations on Wallerian degeneration in explant cultures of cat sciatic nerve. *Journal of Neurocytology*, **15**, 471–82.

Crepel, F. (1982). Regression of functional synapses in the immature mammalian cerebellum. *Trends in Neuroscience*, **5**, 266–70.

Crepel, F., Mariani, J. & Delhaye Bouchaud, N. (1976). Evidence for a multiple innervation of Purkinje cells by climbing fibres in the immature rat cerebellum. *Journal of Neurobiology*, **7**, 567–78.

Cynader, M. & Mitchell, D.E. (1980). Prolonged sensitivity to monocular deprivation in dark reared cats. *Journal of Neurophysiology*, **43**, 1026–40.

Dahm, L.M. & Landmesser, L.T. (1988). The regulation of intramuscular nerve branching during normal development and following activity blockade. *Developmental Biology*, **130**, 621–44.

Daniloff, J.K., Levi, G., Grumet, M., Rieger, F. & Edelman, G.M. (1986). Altered expression of neuronal cell adhesion molecule induced by nerve injury and repair. *Journal of Cell Biology*, **103**, 929–45.

Davey, B., Younkin, L.H. & Younkin, S.G. (1979). Neural control of skeletal muscle cholinesterase: a study using organ cultured rat muscle. *Journal of Physiology*, **289**, 501–15.

Davies, A.M. (1987). Molecular and cellular aspects of patterning sensory neurone connections in the vertebrate nervous system. *Development*, **101**, 185–208.

Davies, A.M., Thoenen, H. & Barde, Y.A. (1986). Different factors from the central nervous system and periphery regulate the survival of sensory neurons. *Nature*, **319**, 497–9.

Davies, J., Cook, G.M.W., Stern, C.D. & Keynes, R.J. (1990). Isolation from chick somites of a glycoprotein fraction which causes collapse of dorsal root ganglion growth cones. *Neuron*, **4**, 11–20.

Davis, H.L. & Heinicke, E.A. (1984). Prevention of denervation atrophy in muscle: mammalian neurotrophic factor is not transferrin. *Brain Research*, **309**, 293–8.

Davis, M.R., Constantine-Paton, M. & Schorr, D. (1983). Dorsal root ganglion removal in *Rana pipiens* produces fewer motor neurons. *Brain Research*, **265**, 282–8.

Dawson, N.J., Hellon, R.F., Herington, J.G. & Young, A.A. (1982). Facial thermal input in the caudal trigeminal nucleus of rats reared at 30° C. *Journal of Physiology*, **333**, 545–54.

Denis-Donini, S. (1989). Expression of dopaminergic phenotypes in the mouse olfactory bulb induced by the calcitonin gene-related peptide. *Nature*, **339**, 701–3.

Dennis, M.J. & Sargent, P.B. (1979). Loss of extrasynaptic ACh sensitivity upon reinnervation of parasympathetic ganglion cells. *Journal of Physiology*, **289**, 263–75.

Dennis, M.J. & Yip, J.W. (1978). Formation and elimination of foreign synapses on adult salamander muscle. *Journal of Physiology*, **274**, 299–310.

Devor, M. & Claman, D. (1980). Mapping and plasticity of acid phosphatase afferents in the rat dorsal horn. *Brain Research*, **190**, 17–28.

Devor, M., Schonfeld, D., Seltzer, Z. & Wall, P.D. (1979). Two modes of cutaneous reinnervation following peripheral nerve injury. *Journal of Comparative Neurology*, **185**, 211–20.

Devor, M. & Wall, P.D. (1981). Plasticity in the spinal cord sensory map following peripheral nerve injury in rats. *Journal of Neuroscience*, **1**, 679–84.

Diamond, J., Coughlin, M., MacIntyre, L., Holmes, M. & Visheau, B. (1987). Evidence that endogenous β nerve growth factor is responsible for the collateral sprouting, but not the regeneration, of nociceptive axons in adult rats. *Proceedings of the National Academy of Science U.S.A.*, **84**, 6596–600.

Diamond, J., Holmes, M. & Visheau, B. (1988). NGF-regulated plasticity in the adult nervous system. *Society of Neuroscience Abstract*, **14**, Part 1, 605.

Diamond, J. & Miledi, R. (1962). A study of foetal and new born rat muscle fibres. *Journal of Physiology*, **162**, 393–408.

Dixon, J.E. & Kintner, C.R. (1989). Cellular contacts required for neural induction in *Xenopus* embryos: evidence for two signals. *Development*, **106**, 749–57.

Dodd, J. & Jessell, T.M. (1988). Axon guidance and the patterning of neuronal projections in vertebrates. *Science*, **242**, 692–9.

Doe, C.Q. & Goodman, C.S. (1985). Early events in insect neurogenesis. II. The role of cell interactions and cell lineage in the determination of neuronal precursor cells. *Developmental Biology*, **111**, 206–19.

Doe, C.Q., Hiromi, Y., Gehring, W.J. & Goodman, C.S. (1988). Expression and function of the segmentation gene fushitarazu during *Drosophila* neurogenesis. *Science*, **239**, 170–5.

Doe, C.Q. & Scott, M.P. (1988). Segmentation and homeotic gene function in the developing nervous system of *Drosophila*. *Trends in Neurosciences*, **11**, 101–6.

Dohrmann, U., Edgar, D., Sendtner, M. & Thoenen, H. (1986). Muscle-derived factors that support survival and promote fibre outgrowth from embryonic chick spinal motor neurons in culture. *Developmental Biology*, **118**, 209–21.

Dohrmann, U., Edgar, D. & Thoenen, H. (1987). Distinct neurotrophic factors from skeletal muscle and the central nervous system interact synergistically to support the survival of cultured embryonic spinal motor neurons. *Developmental Biology*, **124**, 145–52.

Dolphin, A.C., Errington, M.L. & Bliss, R.V.P. (1982). Long-term potentiation of the perforant path in vivo is associated with increased glutamate release. *Nature*, **297**, 496–8.

Dostrovsky, J.O., Jabbur, S. & Millar, J. (1978). Neurons in cat gracile nucleus with both local and widefield inputs. *Journal of Physiology*, **278**, 365–75.

Dostrovsky, J.O., Millar, J. & Wall, P.D. (1976). The immediate shift of afferent drive of dorsal column nucleus cells following deafferentation: a comparison of acute and chronic deafferentation in gracile nucleus and spinal cord. *Experimental Neurology*, **52**, 480–95.

Doucette, R. & Diamond, J. (1987). Normal and precocious sprouting of heat nociceptors in the skin of adult rats. *Journal of Comparative Neurology*, **261**, 592–603.

Doupe, A.J., Patterson, P.H. & Landis, S.C. (1985). Environmental influences in the development of neural crest derivatives: glucocorticoids, growth factors and chromaffin cell plasticity. *Journal of Neuroscience*, **5**, 2119–42.

Dreyer, D., Lagrange, A., Grothe, C. & Unsicker, K. (1989). Basic fibroblast growth factor prevents ontogenetic neuron death in vivo. *Neuroscience Letters*, **99**, 35–8.

Droz, B. (1979). How axonal transport contributes to maintenance of the myelin sheath. *Trends in Neurosciences*, **2**, 146–8.

Duband, J.L., Dufour, S., Hatta, K., Takeichi, M., Edelman, G. & Thiery, J.P. (1987). Adhesion molecules during somitogenesis in the avian embryo. *Journal of Cell Biology*, **104**, 1361–74.

Dubin, M.W., Stark, L.A. & Archer, S.M. (1986). A role for action-potential activity in the development of neuronal connections in the kitten retinogeniculate pathway. *Journal of Neuroscience*, **6**, 1021–36.

Duchen, L. & Strich, S. (1968). The effects of botulinum toxin on the pattern of innervation of skeletal muscle of the mouse. *Quarterly Journal of Experimental Physiology*, **53**, 84–9.

Dunn, P.M. & Marshall, L.M. (1985). Lack of nicotine supersensitivity in frog sympathetic neurones following denervation. *Journal of Physiology*, **363**, 211–25.

Dunwiddie, T. & Lynch, G. (1978). Long-term potentiation and depression of synaptic responses in the rat hippocampus: localisation and frequency dependency. *Journal of Physiology*, **276**, 353–67.

Duxson, M.J. (1982). The effect of post synaptic block on development of the neuromuscular junction in postnatal rats. *Journal of Neurocytology*, **11**, 395–408.

Ebendal, T. & Jacobson, C.O. (1977). Tissue explants affecting extension and orientation of axons in cultured chick embryo ganglia. *Experimental Cell Research*, **105**, 379–87.

Ebendal, T., Olson, L., Seiger, A. & Hedlund, K. O. (1980). Nerve growth factors in the rat iris. *Nature*, **286**, 25–7.

Edgar, D. (1989). Neuronal laminin receptors. *Trends in Neurosciences*, **12**, 248–51.

Edmondson, J.C., Liem, R.K.H., Kuster, J.E. & Hatten, M.E. (1988). Astrotactin: a novel neuronal cell surface antigen that mediates neuron–astroglial interactions in cerebellar microcultures. *Journal of Cell Biology*, **106**, 505–17.

Edstrøm, L. & Kugelberg, E. (1968). Histochemical composition, distribution of fibres and fatiguability of single motor units. *Journal of Neurology, Neurosurgery and Psychiatry*, **31**, 424–33.

English, K.B., Burgess, P.R. & Norman, D.K. (1980). Development of rat Merkel cells. *Journal of Comparative Neurology*, **194**, 475–96.

Farel, P.B. & Bemelmans, S.E. (1985). Specificity of motorneuron projection patterns during development of the bullfrog tadpole. *Journal of Comparative Neurology*, **238**, 128–34.

Fawcett, J.W. (1981). How axons grow down the *Xenopus* optic nerve. *Journal of Embryology and Experimental Morphology*, **65**, 219–33.

Fawcett, J.W., Rokos, J. & Bakst, I. (1989). Oligodendrocytes repel axons and cause axonal growth cone collapse. *Journal of Cell Science*, **92**, 93–100.

Fawcett, J.W. & Willshaw, D.J. (1982). Compound eyes project stripes on the optic tectum in *Xenopus*. *Nature*, **296**, 350–2.

Fifkova, E. & Van Harreveld, A. (1977). Long-lasting morphological changes in dendritic spines of dentate granular cells following stimulation of the entorhinal area. *Journal of Neurocytology*, **6**, 211–30.

Frail, D.E., Musil, L.S., Buonanro, A. & Merlie, J.P. (1989). Expression of RAPsyn (H³K protein) and nicotic acetycholine receptor genes is not coordinately regulated in mouse muscle. *Neuron*, **2**, 1077–86.

Frank, E. (1973). Matching of facilitation at the neuromuscular junction of the lobsters: a possible case for influence of muscle on nerve. *Journal of Physiology*, **223**, 635–58.

(1974). The sensitivity to glutamate of denervated muscles of the crayfish. *Journal of Physiology*, **242**, 371–82.

Fraser, S., Keynes, R. & Lumsden, A. (1990). Segments in the chick embryo hindbrain are defined by cell lineage restrictions. *Nature*, **344**, 431–5.

Freeman, J.A. (1977). Possible regulatory function of acetylcholine receptor in maintenance of retinotectal synapses. *Nature*, **269**, 218–22.

Freeman, R.D. & Ohzawa, I. (1988). Monocularly deprived cats : binocular tests of cortical cells reveal functional connections from the deprived eye. *Journal of Neuroscience*, **8**, 2491–506.

Fregnac, Y. & Imbert, M. (1984). Development of neuronal selectivity in primary visual cortex of cat. *Physiological Reviews*, **64**, 325–434.

Friede, R.L. (1972). Control of myelin formation by axon caliber (with a model of the control mechanism). *Journal of Comparative Neurology*, **144**, 233–52.

Friede, R.L. & Bischhausen, R. (1980). The fine structure of stumps of transected nerve fibers in subserial sections. *Journal of Neurological Science*, **44**, 181–203.

Fujisawa, H. (1981). Retinotopic analysis of fibre pathways in the regenerating retinotectal system of the adult newt *Cynops pyrrhyogaster*. *Brain Research*, **206**, 27–37.

Furber, S., Oppenheim, R.W. & Prevette, D. (1987). Naturally-occurring neuron death in the ciliary ganglion of the chick embryo following removal of preganglionic input: evidence for the role of afferents in ganglion cell survival. *Journal of Neuroscience*, **7**, 1816–32.

Gaze, R.M. (1974). Neuronal specificity. *British Medical Bulletin*, **30**, 116–21.

Gaze, R.M., Keating, M.J., Ostberg, A. & Chung, S. H. (1979). The relationship between retinal and tectal growth in larval *Xenopus*: implications for the development of the retinotectal projection. *Journal of Embryology and Experimental Morphology*, **53**, 103–43.

Gerding, R., Robbins, N. & Antosiak, J. (1977). Efficiency of reinnervation of neonatal rat muscle by original and foreign nerves. *Developmental Biology*, **61**, 177–83.

Gilbert, P.F.C. (1974). A theory of memory that explains the function and structure of the cerebellum. *Brain Research*, **70**, 1–18.

Gilbert, P.F.C. & Thach, W.T. (1977). Purkinje cell activity during motor learning. *Brain Research*, **128**, 309–28.

Ghysen, A. & Dambly-Chaudiere, C. (1989). Genesis of the *Drosophila* peripheral nervous system. *Trends in Genetics*, **5**, 251–5.

Glaze, K.A. & Turner, J.E. (1978). Regenerative repair in the severed optic nerve of the newt (*Triturus viridescens*): effect of nerve growth factor antiserum. *Experimental Neurology*, **58**, 500–10.

Glicksman, M.A. & Sanes, J.R. (1983). Differentiation of motor nerve terminals formed in the absence of muscle fibres. *Journal of Neurocytology*, **12**, 666–77.

Globus, A. & Scheibel, A.B. (1967). Pattern and field in cortical structure: the rabbit. *Journal of Comparative Neurology*, **131**, 55–72.

Goh, J.W. & Pennefather, P.S. (1989). A pertussis toxin-sensitive G protein in hippocampal long-term potentiation. *Science*, **244**, 980–3.

Goldberger, M.E. (1977). Locomotor recovery after unilateral hindlimb deafferentation. *Brain Research*, **123**, 59–74.

Goldberger, M.E. & Murray, M. (1982). Lack of sprouting and its presence after lesions of the cat spinal cord. *Brain Research*, **241**, 227–39.

Goodman, C.S. (1978). Isogenic grasshoppers: genetic variability in the morphology of identified neurons. *Journal of Comparative Neurology*, **182**, 681–705.

Goodman, C.S. & Bastiani, M.J. (1984). How embryonic nerve cells recognise one another. *Scientific American*, **251**(6), 50–8.

Goodman, C.S. & Bate, M. (1981). Neuronal development of the grasshopper. *Trends in Neurosciences*, **4**, 163–9.

Gordon-Weeks, P.R. (1988). RNA transport in dendrites. *Trends in Neurosciences*, **11**, 342–3.

Gordon, H. & Van Essen, D.C. (1985). Specific innervation of muscle fibre types in a developmentally polyinnervated muscle. *Developmental Biology*, **111**, 42–50.

Gordon, T., Perry, R., Tuffery, A.R. & Vrbova, G. (1974). Possible mechanisms determining synapse formation in developing skeletal muscles of the chick. *Cell Tissue Research*, **155**, 13–25.

Gorin, P.D. & Johnson, E.M. (1980). Effects of long term NGF deprivation on the nervous system of the adult rat: an experimental autoimmune approach. *Brain Research*, **198**, 27–42.

Gorza, L., Gundersen, K., Lømo, T., Schiaffino, S. & Westgaard, R. H. (1988). Slow-to-fast transformation of denervated soleus muscles by chronic high-frequency stimulation in the rat. *Journal of Physiology*, **402**, 627–49.

Goslin, K. & Banker, G.A. (1989). Experimental observations on the development of polarity by hippocampal neurones in culture. *Journal of Cell Biology*, **188**, 1507–16.

Goslin, K., Schreyer, D.J., Skene, J.H.P. & Banker, G. (1988). Development of neuronal polarity: GAP-43 distinguishes axonal from dendritic growth cones. *Nature*, **336**, 672–4.

Govind, C.K. & Kent, K.S. (1982). Transformation of fast fibres to slow prevented by lack of activity in developing lobster muscle. *Nature*, **298**, 755–7.

Greenwald, I. (1989). Cell-cell interactions that specify certain cell fates in *C. elegans* development. *Trends in Genetics*, **5**, 237–41.

Greuel, J.M., Luhmann, H.J. & Singer, W. (1988). Pharmacological induction of use-dependent receptive field modifications in the visual cortex. *Science*, **242**, 74–7.

Grimm, C.M. (1971). An evaluation of myotypic respecification in axolotls. *Journal of Experimental Zoology*, **178**, 479–96.

Grinnell, A.D., Letinsky, M.S. & Rheuben, M.B. (1979). Competitive interaction between foreign nerves innervating frog skeletal muscle. *Journal of Physiology*, **289**, 241–62.

Guillery, R.W. (1972). Binocular competition in the control of geniculate cell growth. *Journal of Comparative Neurology*, **144**, 117–30.

(1973). The effect of lid suture upon the growth of cells in the dorsal lateral geniculate nucleus of kittens. *Journal of Comparative Neurology*, **148**, 417–22.

Gundersen, R.W. & Barrett, J.N. (1980). Characteristics of the turning response of dorsal root neurites towards NGF. *Journal of Cell Biology*, **87**, 546–54.

Gustafsson, B. & Wigstrom, H. (1988). Physiological mechanisms underlying long-term potentiation. *Trends in Neurosciences*, **11**, 156–62.

Gutmann, E. (1945). Reinnervation of muscle by sensory nerve fibres. *Journal of Anatomy*, **79**, 1–8.

Halfter, W., Chiquet Ehrismann, R. & Tucker, R.P. (1989). The effect of tenascin and embryonic basal lamina on the behavior and morphology of neural crest cells in vitro. *Developmental Biology*, **132**, 14–25.

Hamburger, V. (1980). Trophic interactions in neurogenesis: a personal historical account. *Annual Review of Neuroscience*, **3**, 269–78.

Hamburger, V., Brunso Bechtold, J.L. & Yip, J.W. (1981). Neuronal death in the spinal ganglia of the chick embryo and its reduction by nerve growth factor. *Journal of Neuroscience*, **1**, 60–71.

Hamburger, V. & Levi-Montalcini, R. (1949). Proliferation, differentiation and degeneration in the spinal ganglia of the chick embryo under normal and experimental conditions. *Journal of Experimental Zoology*, **111**, 457–507.

Hamburger, V. & Oppenheim, R.W. (1982). Naturally occurring neuronal death in vertebrates. *Neuroscience Commentaries*, **1**, 39–55.

Hanley, M.R. (1989). Mitogenic neurotransmitters. *Nature*, **340**, 97.

Hardman, V.J. & Brown, M.C. (1987). Accuracy of re-innervation of rat intercostal muscles by their own segmental nerves. *Journal of Neuroscience*, **7**, 1031–6.

Harrelson, A.L. & Goodman, C.S. (1988). Growth cone guidance in insects: Fasciclin II is a member of the immunoglobulin superfamily. *Science*, **242**, 700–8.

Harris, W.A. (1989). Local positional cues in the neuroepithelium guide retinal axons in embryonic *Xenopus* brain. *Nature*, **339**, 218–20.

Harris, W.A., Holt, C.E. & Bonhoeffer, F. (1987). Retinal axons with and without their somata, growing to and arborizing in the tectum of Xenopus embryos: a time-lapse video study of single fibres in vivo. *Development*, **101**, 123–33.

Harrison, R.G. (1908). Embryonic transplantation and development of the nervous system. *Anatomical Record*, **2**, 385–410.

(1910). The outgrowth of the nerve fibre as a mode of protoplasmic movement. *Journal of Experimental Zoology*, **9**, 787–846.

Hatta, K., Takagi, S., Fujisawa, H. & Takeichi, M. (1987). Spatial and temporal expression pattern of N-cadherin adhesion molecules correlated with morphogenetic processes of chicken embryos. *Developmental Biology*, **120**, 215–27.

Hatten, M.E. & Mason, C.A. (1986). Neuron-astroglia interactions in vitro and in vivo. *Trends in Neurosciences*, **9**, 168–74.

Hawkins, R.D., Castellucci, V.F. & Kandel, E.R. (1981). Interneurons involved in mediation and modulation of the gill-withdrawal reflex in *Aplysia*. II. Identified neurons produce heterosynaptic facilitation contributing to behavioural sensitization. *Journal of Neurophysiology*, **45**, 315–26.

Hayes, W.P. & Meyer, R.L. (1988). Retinotopically inappropriate synapses of subnormal density formed by surgically misdirected optic fibres in goldfish tectum. *Developmental Brain Research*, **38**, 304–12.

Haynes, L.W. & Smith, M.E. (1982). Selective inhibition of motor endplate specific acetylcholinesterase by β-endorphin and related peptides. *Neuroscience*, **7**, 1007–13.

Haynes, L.W., Smyth, D.G. & Zakarian, S. (1982). Immunocytochemical localisation of β-endorphin (lipotropin c-fragment) in the developing rat spinal cord and hypothalamus. *Brain Research*, **232**, 115–28.

Hebb, D.O. (1949). *The Organisation of Behaviour*. New York, John Wiley.

Heidemann, M.K. (1977). Neurophysiological and behavioural evidence for selective reinnervation of skin grafted *Rana pipiens*. *Proceedings of National Academy of Science U.S.A*, **74**, 5749–53.

Henderson, C.E. (1988). The role of muscle in the development and differentiation of spinal motor neurons : in vitro studies. *Ciba Foundation Symposium*, **138**, 172–91.

Hendry, I.H., Iversen, L.L. & Black, I.B. (1973). A comparison of the neural regulation of tyrosine hydroxylase activity in sympathetic ganglia of adult mice and rats. *Journal of Neurochemistry*, **20**, 1683–9.

Herrera, A.A. & Grinnell, A.D. (1981). Contralateral denervation causes enhanced transmitter release from frog motor nerve terminals. *Nature*, **291**, 495–7.

Herrera, A.A., Grinnell, A.D. & Wolowske, B. (1985). Ultrastructural correlates of experimentally altered transmitter release efficacy in frog motor nerve terminals. *Neuroscience*, **16**, 491–500.

Herrera, A.A. & Scott, D.R. (1985). Motor axon sprouting in frog sartorius muscle is not altered by contralateral axotomy. *Journal of Neurocytology*, **14**, 145–56.

Heumann, R. (1987). Regulation of the synthesis of nerve growth factor. *Journal of Experimental Biology*, **132**, 133–50.

Heumann, R., Korsching, S., Scott, J. & Thoenen, H. (1984). Relationship between levels of nerve growth factor (NGF) and its messenger RNA in sympathetic ganglia and peripheral target tissues. *EMBO Journal*, **3**, 3183–9.

Hirsch, V.B. & Spinelli, D.N. (1971). Modification of the distribution of receptive field orientation in cats by selective visual exposure during development. *Experimental Brain Research*, **12**, 509–27.

Hofer, M.M. & Barde, Y.A. (1988). Brain-derived neurotrophic factor prevents neuronal death in vivo. *Nature*, **331**, 261–2.

Hoffman, P.N. (1988). Distinct roles of neurofilament and tubulin gene expression in axonal growth. *Ciba Foundation Symposium*, **138**, 192–200.

Hoffmann, H. (1950). Local re-innervation in partially denervated muscle : a histo-physiological study. *Australian Journal of Experimental Biological Sciences*, **28**, 383–97.

Hollenbeck, P.J. & Bray, D. (1987). Rapidly transported organelles containing membrane and cytoskeletal components: their relation to axonal growth. *Journal of Cell Biology*, **105**, 2827–35.

Hollyday, M. (1981). Rules of motor innervation in chick embryos with supernumerary limbs. *Journal of Comparative Neurology*, **202**, 439–65.

Hollyday, M. & Hamburger, V. (1976). Reduction in naturally occurring motor neuron loss by enlargement of the periphery. *Journal of Comparative Neurology*, **170**, 311–20.

Holt, C.E. (1984). Does timing of axon outgrowth influence initial retinotectal topography in *Xenopus? Journal of Neuroscience*, **4**, 1130–52.

Honig, M.G. (1982). The development of sensory projection patterns in embryonic chick hind limbs. *Journal of Physiology*, **330**, 175–202.

Hope, R.A., Hammond, B.J. & Gaze, R.M. (1976). The arrow model: retinotectal specificity and map formation in the goldfish visual system. *Proceedings of the Royal Society of London*, B**194**, 447–66.

Hopkins, W.G., Brown, M.C. & Keynes, R.J. (1981). Nerve growth from nodes of Ranvier in inactive muscle. *Brain Research*, **222**, 125–8.

Hosley, M.A., Hughes, S.E. & Oakley, B. (1987). Neural induction of taste buds. *Journal of Comparative Neurology*, **260**, 224–32.

Hoy, R.R., Bittner, G.D. & Kennedy, D. (1967). Regeneration in crustacean motor neurons: evidence for axonal fusion. *Science*, **156**, 251–3.

Hubel, D.H. (1982). Exploration of the primary visual cortex, 1955–1978. *Nature*, **299**, 515–24.

Hubel, D.H. & Wiesel, T.N. (1963). Receptive fields in striate cortex of very young, visually inexperienced kittens. *Journal of Neurophysiology*, **26**, 994–1002.

(1965). Binocular interaction in striate cortex of kittens reared with artificial squint. *Journal of Neurophysiology*, **28**, 1041–59.

(1970). The period of susceptibility to the physiological effects of unilateral eye closure in kittens. *Journal of Physiology*, **206**, 419–36.

(1979). Brain mechanisms of vision. *Scientific American*, **241**, 130–45.

Hubel, D.H., Wiesel, T.N. & Le Vay, S. (1977). Plasticity of ocular dominance columns in monkey striate cortex. *Philosophical Transactions of the Royal Society of London*, B**278**, 377–404.

Hume, R.I. & Purves, D. (1981). Geometry of neonatal neurones and the regulation of synapse elimination. *Nature*, **293**, 469–71.

Hunter, D.D., Shah, V., Merlie, J.P. & Sanes, J.R. (1989). A laminin-like adhesive protein concentrated in the synaptic cleft of the neuromuscular junction. *Nature*, **338**, 229–33.

Hynes, R.O. (1987). Integrins: a family of cell surface receptors. *Cell*, **48**, 549–54.

Ignatius, M.J. & Reichardt, L.F. (1988). Identification and characterization of a neuronal laminin receptor: an integrin heterodimer binding laminin in a cation-dependent manner. *Neuron*, **1**, 713–25.

Ignatius, M.J., Shooter, E.M., Pitas, R.E. & Mahley, R.W. (1987). Lipoprotein uptake by neuronal growth cones in vitro. *Science*, **236**, 959–62.

Innocenti, G.M. (1981). Growth and reshaping of axons in the establishment of visual callosal connections. *Science*, **212**, 824–7.

Ishii, D.N. (1989). Relationship of insulin-like growth factor II gene expression in muscle to synaptogenesis. *Proceedings of the National Academy of Science U.S.A.*, **86**, 2898–902.

Ito, M., Sakurai, M. & Tongroach, P. (1982). Climbing fibre induced depression of both mossy fibre responsiveness and glutamate sensitivity of cerebellar Purkinje cells. *Journal of Physiology*, **324**, 113–34.

Jackson, P.C. (1983). Reduced activity during development delays the normal rearrangement of synapses in the rabbit ciliary ganglion. *Journal of Physiology*, **345**, 319–27.

Jackson, P.C. & Diamond, J. (1983). Failure of intact cutaneous mechanosensory axons to sprout functional collaterals in skin of adult rabbits. *Brain Research*, **273**, 277–84.

Jacobs, J.R. & Goodman, C.S. (1989). Embryonic development of axon pathways in the *Drosophila* CNS.1. A glial scaffold appears before first growth cones. *Journal of Neuroscience*, **9**, 2402–11.

Jaffe, L.F. & Poo, M.M. (1979). Neurites grow faster towards the cathode than the anode in a steady field. *Journal of Experimental Zoology*, **209**, 115–28.

Jansen, J.K.S., Lømo, T., Nicolaysen, T. & Westgaard, R.H. (1973). Hyperinnervation of skeletal muscle fibres: dependence on muscle activity. *Science*, **181**, 559–61.

Jeffery, G. (1989). Distribution and trajectory of uncrossed axons in the optic nerves of pigmented and albino rats. *Journal of Comparative Neurology*, **289**, 462–6.

Jeffery, G. & Perry, V.H. (1982). Evidence for ganglion cell death during development of the ipsilateral retinal projection in the rat. *Developmental Brain Research*, **2**, 176–80.

Jenq, C.B., Chung, K. & Coggeshall, R.E. (1986). Postnatal loss of axons in normal rat sciatic nerve. *Journal of Comparative Neurology*, **244**, 445–50.

Jessell, T.M. (1988). Adhesion molecules and the hierarchy of neural development. *Neuron*, **1**, 3–13.

Jessen, K.R., Mirsky, R. & Morgan, L. (1987). Myelinated but not unmyelinated axons reversibly down-regulate N-CAM in Schwann cells. *Journal of Neurocytology*, **16**, 681–8.

Johnson, E.M., Gorin, P.D., Brandeis, L.D. & Pearson, J. (1980). Dorsal root ganglion neurons are destroyed by exposure in utero to maternal antibody to nerve growth factor. *Science*, **210**, 916–8.

Johnson, E.M., Taniuchi, M. & Di Stefano, P.S. (1988). Expression and possible function of nerve growth factor receptors on Schwann cells. *Trends in Neurosciences*, **11**, 299–304.

Jones, R. & Vrbova, G. (1974). Two factors responsible for the development of denervation hypersensitivity. *Journal of Physiology*, **236**, 517P.

Jones, S.P., Ridge, R.M.A.P. & Rowlerson, A. (1987a). The non-selective innervation of muscle fibres and mixed composition of motor units in a muscle of neonatal rat. *Journal of Physiology*, **386**, 377–94.

(1987b). Rat muscle during postnatal development: evidence in favour of no interconversion between fast- and slow-twitch fibres. *Journal of Physiology*, **386**, 395–406.

Jones, W.H. & Thomas, D.B. (1962). Changes in the dendritic organization of neurons in the cerebral cortex following deafferentation. *Journal of Anatomy*, **96**, 375–81.

Jordan, C.L., Letinsky, M.S. & Arnold, A.P. (1989a). The role of gonadal hormones in neuromuscular synapse elimination in rats. I. Androgen delays the loss of multiple innervation in the levator ani muscle. *Journal of Neuroscience*, **9**, 229–38.

(1989b). The role of gonadal hormones in neuromuscular synapse elimination in rats. II. Multiple innervation persists in the adult levator ani muscle after juvenile androgen treatment. *Journal of Neuroscience*, **9**, 239–47.

Kandel, E.R. & Schwartz, J.H. (1982). Molecular biology of an elementary form of learning: modulation of transmitter release through cyclic AMP-dependent protein kinase. *Science*, **218**, 433–43.

Kasamatsu, T. & Pettigrew, J.D. (1976). Depletion of brain catecholamines: failure of ocular dominance shift after monocular occlusion in kittens. *Science*, **194**, 206–9.

Katz, M.J. & Lasek, R.J. (1978). Eyes transplanted to tadpole tails send axons rostrally in two spinal cord tracts. *Science*, **199**, 202–3.

Katz, M.J., Lasek, R.J. & Nauta, H.J.W. (1980). Ontogeny of substrate pathways and the origin of the neural circuit pattern. *Neuroscience*, **5**, 821–33.

Kauer, J.A., Malenka, R.C. & Nicoll, R.A. (1988). A persistent postsynaptic modification mediates long-term potentiation in the hippocampus. *Neuron*, **1**, 911–17.

Keating, M.J. (1974). The role of visual function in the patterning of binocular visual connections. *British Medical Bulletin*, **30**, 145–51.

Keynes, R.J. (1987). Schwann cells during neural development and regeneration: leaders or followers? *Trends in Neurosciences*, **10**, 137–9.

Keynes, R.J. & Lumsden, A. (1990). Segmentation and the origin of regional diversity in the vertebrate central nervous system. *Neuron*, **4**, 1–9.

Keynes, R.J., Hopkins, W.G. & Brown, M.C. (1983). Sprouting of mammalian motor neurones at nodes of Ranvier: the role of the denervated motor endplate. *Brain Research*, **264**, 209–13.

Keynes, R.J. & Stern, C.D. (1988). Mechanisms of vertebrate segmentation. *Development*, **103**, 413–29.

Keynes, R.J., Stirling, R.V., Stern, C.D. & Summerbell, D. (1987). The specificity of motor innervation of the chick wing does not depend upon the segmental origin of muscles. *Development*, **99**, 565–75.

Kimmel, C.B. (1982). Development of synapses on the Mauthner neuron. *Trends in Neuroscience*, **5**, 47–50.

Kinnamon, E. & Aldskogius, H. (1986). Collateral sprouting of sensory axons in the glabrous skin of the hindpaw after chronic sciatic nerve lesions in adult and neonatal rats: a morphological study. *Brain Research*, **377**, 73–82.

Klein, M., Shapiro, E. & Kandel, E.R. (1980). Synaptic plasticity and the modulation of the Ca^{2+} current. *Journal of Experimental Biology*, **89**, 117–57.

Kleinschmidt, A., Bear, M.F. & Singer, W. (1987). Blockade of 'NMDA' receptors disrupts experience dependent plasticity of kitten striate cortex. *Science*, **238**, 355–8.

Knudsen, E.I., Knudsen, P.F. & Esterly, S.D. (1982). Early auditory experience modifies sound localisation in barn owls. *Nature*, **295**, 238–40.

Konishi, M. & Gurney, M.E. (1982). Sexual differentiation of brain and behaviour. *Trends in Neuroscience*, **5**, 20–3.

Koppel, H. & Innocenti, G.M. (1983). Is there a genuine exuberancy of callosal projections in development? A quantitative EM study in the cat. *Neuroscience Letters*, **41**, 33–40.

Korneliussen, H. & Jansen, J.K.S. (1976). Morphological aspects of the elimination of polyneuronal innervation of skeletal muscle fibres in newborn rats. *Journal of Neurocytology*, **5**, 591–604.

Kuffler, D.P., Thompson, W. & Jansen, J.K.S. (1980). The fate of foreign endplates in cross innervated rat soleus muscle. *Proceedings of the Royal Society of London*, **B208**, 189–222.

Kuffler, S.W., Dennis, M.J. & Harris, A.J. (1971). The development of chemosensitivity in extra synaptic areas of the neuronal surface after denervation of parasympathetic ganglion cells in the heart of the frog. *Proceedings of the Royal Society of London*, **B177**, 555–63.

Kuromi, H., Gonoi, T. & Hosegawa, S. (1979). Partial purification and characterisation of neurotrophic substance affecting tetrodotoxin sensitivity of organ cultured mouse muscle. *Brain Research*, **175**, 109–18.

Laing, N.G. & Prestige, M.C. (1978). Prevention of spontaneous motor neurone death in chick embryos. *Journal of Physiology*, **282**, 33P.

Lamb, A.H. (1976). The projection patterns of the ventral horn to the hind limb during development. *Developmental Biology*, **54**, 82–99.

(1977). Neuronal death in the development of the somatotopic projections of the ventral horn in *Xenopus*. *Brain Research*, **134**, 145–50.

(1980). Motoneurone counts in Xenopus frogs reared with one bilaterally innervated hind limb. *Nature*, **284**, 347–50.

(1981). Selective bilateral motor innervation in *Xenopus* tadpoles with one hindlimb. *Journal of Embryology and Experimental Morphology*, **65**, 149–63.

Lamb, A.H., Ferns, M.J. & Klose, K. (1989). Peripheral competition in the control of sensory neuron numbers in *Xenopus* frogs reared with a single bilaterally innervated hindlimb. *Developmental Brain Research*, **45**, 149–53.

Lamborghini, J.E. (1980). Rohon-Beard cells and other large neurons in *Xenopus* embryos originate during gastrulation. *Journal of Comparative Neurology*, **189**, 323–33.

LaMotte, C.C., Kapodia, S.E. & Kocol, C.M. (1989). Deafferentation-induced expansion of saphenous terminal field labelling in the adult dorsal horn following pronase injection of the sciatic nerve. *Journal of Comparative Neurology*, **288**, 311–25.

Lance-Jones, C. (1988). Development of neuromuscular connections: guidance of motor neuron axons to muscles in the embryonic chick hindlimb. *Ciba Foundation Symposium*, **138**, 97–115.

Lance-Jones, C. & Landmesser, L. (1980). Motoneurone projection patterns in the chick hind limb following early partial reversals of the spinal cord. *Journal of Physiology*, **302**, 581–602.

  (1982). Pathway selection by chick lumbosacral motor neurons in an experimentally altered environment. *Proceedings of the Royal Society of London*, **B214**, 19–52.

Land, P.W. & Lund, R.D. (1979). Development of the rat's uncrossed retinotectal pathway and its relation to plasticity studies. *Science*, **205**, 698–700.

Lander, A.D. (1989). Understanding the molecules of neural cell contacts: Emerging patterns of structure and function. *Trends in Neurosciences*, **12**, 189–95.

Landmesser, L. (1971). Contractile and electrical responses of vagus-innervated frog sartorius muscles. *Journal of Physiology*, **213**, 707–25.

  (1972). Pharmacological properties, cholinesterase activity and anatomy of nerve muscle junctions in vagus innervated frog sartorius. *Journal of Physiology*, **220**, 243–56.

  (1978). The development of motor projection patterns in the chick hind limb. *Journal of Physiology*, **284**, 391–414.

  (1984). The development of specific motor pathways in the chick embryo. *Trends in Neurosciences*, **7**, 336–9.

Landmesser, L., Dahm, L., Schultz, K. & Rutishauser, U. (1988). Distinct roles for adhesion molecules during innervation of embryonic chick muscle. *Developmental Biology*, **130**, 645–70.

Landmesser, L. & Pilar, G. (1976). Fate of ganglionic synapses and ganglion cell axons during normal and induced cell death. *Journal of Cell Biology*, **68**, 357–74.

Langley, J.N. (1897). On the regeneration of pre ganglionic and post ganglionic visceral nerve fibres. *Journal of Physiology*, **22**, 215–30.

Lanser, M.E. & Fallon, J.F. (1984). Development of the brachial lateral motor column in the wingless mutant chick embryo. *Journal of Neuroscience*, **4**, 2043–50.

Lasek, R.J. (1982). Translocation of the neuronal cytoskeleton and axonal locomotion. *Philosophical Transactions of the Royal Society of London*, **B299**, 313–27.

Laskowski, M.B. & High, J.A. (1989). Expression of nerve-muscle topography during development. *Journal of Neuroscience*, **9**, 175–82.

Laskowski, M.B. & Sanes, J.R. (1988). Topographically selective reinnervation of adult mammalian skeletal muscle. *Journal of Neuroscience*, **8**, 3094–9.

Law, M.I. & Constantine-Paton, M. (1981). Anatomy and physiology of experimentally induced striped tecta. *Journal of Neuroscience*, **1**, 741–59.

Le Douarin, N.M. (1982). *The Neural Crest*. Cambridge, Cambridge University Press.

  (1986a). Cell line segregation during peripheral nervous system ontogeny. *Science*, **231**, 1515–22.

  (1986b). Cephalic ectodermal placodes and neurogenesis. *Trends in Neurosciences*, **9**, 175–80.

Le Douarin, N.M. & Teillet, M.A. (1974). Experimental analysis of the migration and differentiation of neuroblasts of the autonomic nervous system and of neurectodermal mesenchymal derivatives using a biological cell marking technique. *Developmental Biology*, **41**, 162–84.

Leistol, I.L., Maehlen, J. & Njå, A. (1986). Selctive synaptic connections: significance of recognition and competition in mature sympathetic ganglion. *Trends in Neurosciences*, **9**, 21–4.

Letourneau, P.C. (1975). Cell to substratum adhesion and guidance of axonal elongation. *Developmental Biology*, **44**, 92–101.

(1979). Cell substratum adhesion of neurite growth cones, and its role in neurite elongation. *Experimental Cell Research*, **124**, 127–38.

(1981). Immunocytochemical evidence for colocalization in neurite growth cones of actin and myosin and their relationship to cell substratum adhesions. *Developmental Biology*, **85**, 113–22.

Levi-Montalcini, R. & Calissano, P. (1979). The Nerve Growth Factor. *Scientific American*, **240**, 44–53.

Levi-Montalcini, R. & Cohen, S. (1960). Effects of the extract of the mouse submaxillary salivary glands on the sympathetic system of mammals. *Annals of the New York Academy of Sciences*, **85**, 324–41.

Levine, R.L. & Jacobson, M. (1975). Discontinuous mapping of retina onto tectum innervated by both eyes. *Brain Research*, **98**, 172–6.

Levitt, P., Cooper, M.L. & Rakic, P. (1981). Co-existence of neuronal and glial precursor cells in the cerebral ventricular zone of the fetal monkey: an ultrastructural immunoperoxidase analysis. *Journal of Neuroscience*, **1**, 27–39.

Lewis, J., Chevallier, A., Kieny, M. & Wolpert, L. (1981). Muscle nerves do not develop in chick wings devoid of muscle. *Journal of Embryology and Experimental Morphology*, **64**, 211–32.

Lewis, P.D. (1968). Mitotic activity in the primate subependymal layer and the genesis of gliomas. *Nature*, **217**, 974–5.

Lichtman, J.W. (1977). The organisation of synaptic connections in the rat submandibular ganglion during postnatal development. *Journal of Physiology*, **273**, 155–78.

Lichtman, J.W. & Purves, D. (1980). The elimination of redundant preganglionic innervation to hamster sympathetic ganglion cells in early postnatal life. *Journal of Physiology*, **301**, 213–28.

Lichtman, J.W., Purves, D. & Yip, J.W. (1979). On the purpose of selective innervation of guinea pig superior cervical ganglion cells. *Journal of Physiology*, **292**, 69–84.

Liesi, P. & Silver, J. (1988). Is astrocyte laminin involved in axon guidance in the mammalian CNS? *Developmental Biology*, **130**, 774–85.

Lillien, L.E., Sendtner, M., Rohrer, H., Hughes, S.M. & Raff, M.C. (1988). Type-2 astrocyte development in rat brain is initiated by a CNTF-like protein produced by Type-1 astrocytes. *Neuron*, **1**, 485–94.

Lincoln, J.S., McCormick, D.A. & Thompson, R.F. (1982). Ipsilateral cerebellar lesions prevent learning of the classically conditioned nictitating membrane/eyelid response. *Brain Research*, **242**, 190–3.

Linden, R. & Perry, V.H. (1982). Ganglion cell death within the developing retina: a regulatory role for retinal dendrites? *Neuroscience*, **7**, 2813–27.

Lindholm, D., Heumann, R., Meyer, M. & Thoenen, H. (1987). Interleukin-1 regulates synthesis of nerve growth factor in non-neuronal cells of the rat sciatic nerve. *Nature*, **330**, 658–9.

Lindsay, R.M. & Harman, A.J. (1989). Nerve growth factor regulates expression of neuropeptide genes in adult sensory neurons. *Nature*, **337**, 362–4.

Liu, C.M. & Chambers, W.W. (1958). Intraspinal sprouting of dorsal root axons. *Archives of Neurology and Psychiatry*, **79**, 46–61.

Loesche, J. & Steward, D. (1977). Behavioural correlates of denervation and reinnervation of the hippocampal formation of the rat: recovery of alternation performance following unilateral entorhinal cortex lesions. *Brain Research Bulletin*, **2**, 21–39.

Lømo, T. (1974). Neurotrophic control of colchicine effects on muscle? *Nature*, **249**, 473–4.

(1980). What controls the development of neuromuscular junctions? *Trends in Neurosciences*, **3**, 126–9.

Lømo, T., Massoulie, J. & Vigny, M. (1985). Stimulation of denervated rat soleus muscle with fast and slow activity patterns induces different expression of acetylcholinesterase molecular forms. *Journal of Neuroscience*, **5**, 1180–7.

Lømo, T., Pockett, S. & Sommerschild, H. (1988). Control of number and distribution of synapses during ectopic synapse formation in adult rat soleus muscle. *Neuroscience*, **24**, 673–80.

Lømo, T. & Rosenthal, J. (1972). Control of acetylcholine sensitivity by muscle activity in the rat. *Journal of Physiology*, **221**, 493–513.

Lømo, T. & Slater, C.R. (1980a). Acetylcholine sensitivity of developing ectopic nerve muscle junctions in adult rat soleus muscles. *Journal of Physiology*, **303**, 173–89.

(1980b). Control of junctional acetylcholinesterase by neural and muscular influences in the rat. *Journal of Physiology*, **303**, 191–202.

Lømo, T. & Westgaard, R.H. (1976). Control of acetylcholine sensitivity in rat muscle fibres. *Cold Spring Harbor Symposia on Quantitative Biology*, **40**, 263–74.

Lømo, T., Westgaard, R.H. & Dahl, R.H. (1974). Contractile properties of muscle: control by pattern of muscle activity in the rat. *Proceedings of the Royal Society of London*, **B187**, 99–103.

Ludwin, S.K. (1984). Proliferation of mature oligodendrocytes after trauma to the central nervous system. *Nature*, **308**, 274–5.

Luenicka, G.A., Blundon, J.A. & Govind, C.K. (1988). Early experience influences the development of bilateral asymmetry in a lobster motor neuron. *Developmental Biology*, **129**, 84–90.

Lukowiak, K. & Colebrook, E. (1988). Classical conditioning alters the efficacy of identified gill motor neurones in producing gill withdrawal movements in *Aplysia*. *Journal of Experimental Biology*, **140**, 273–85.

Lumsden, A. & Keynes, R. (1989). Segmental patterns of neuronal development in the chick hindbrain. *Nature*, **337**, 424–8.

Lumsden, A.G.S. & Davies, A.M. (1983). Earliest sensory nerve fibres are guided to peripheral targets by attractants other than nerve growth factor. *Nature*, **306**, 786–8.

Lund, R.D., Mitchell, D.E. & Henry, G.H. (1978). Squint induced modification of callosal connections in cats. *Brain Research*, **144**, 169–72.

Lundborg, G., Longo, F.M. & Varon, S. (1982). Nerve regeneration model and trophic factors in vivo. *Brain Research*, **232**, 157–61.

Lunn, E.R., Brown, M.C. & Perry, V.H. (1990). The pattern of axonal degeneration in the peripheral nervous system varies with different types of lesion. *Neuroscience*, **35**, 157–65.

Lunn, E.R., Perry, V.H., Brown, M.C., Rosen, H. & Gordon, S. (1989). Absence of Wallerian degeneration does not hinder regeneration in peripheral nerve. *European Journal of Neuroscience*, **1**, 27–33.

Lynch, G., Deadwyler, S. & Cotman, C.W. (1973). Postlesion axonal growth produces permanent functional connections. *Science*, **180**, 1364–6.

Lynch, M.A., Clements, M.P., Errington, M.C. & Bliss, J.V.P. (1988). Increased hydrolysis of phosphatidyl-4, 5-biphosphate in long-term potentiation. *Neuroscience Letters*, **84**, 291–6.

Macagno, E.R., Lopresti, U. & Levinthal, C. (1973). Structure and development of neuronal connections in isogenic organisms: variations and similarities in the optic system of *Daphnia magna*. *Proceedings of the National Academy of Science U.S.A.*, **70**, 57–61.

Maggs, A. & Scholes, J. (1986). Glial domains and nerve fibre patterns in the fish retinotectal pathway. *Journal of Neuroscience*, **6**, 424–43.

Magill-Salc, C. & McMahan, U.J. (1988). Motor neurons contain agrin-like molecules. *Journal of Cell Biology*, **107**, 1825–33.

Malenka, R.C., Kauer, J.A., Perkel, D.J., Mark, M.D., Kelly, P.T., Nicoll, R.A. & Waxham, M.N. (1989). An essential role for postsynaptic calmodulin and protein kinase activity in long-term potentiation. *Nature*, **340**, 554–56.

Mark, R.F. (1965). Fin movement after regeneration of neuromuscular connections: an investigation of myotypic specifity. *Experimental Neurology*, **12**, 292–302.

(1970). Chemospecific synaptic repression as a possible memory store. *Nature*, **225**, 178–9.

Markelonis, G.J. & Oh, T.H. (1979). A sciatic nerve protein has a trophic effect on development and maintenance of skeletal muscle cells in culture. *Proceedings of the National Academy of Science U.S.A.*, **76**, 2470–4.

Markus, H. & Pomeranz, B. (1987). Saphenous has weak ineffective synapses in sciatic territory of rat spinal cord: electrical stimulation of the saphenous and application of drugs reveal these somototopically inappropriate synapses. *Brain Research*, **416**, 315–21.

Marlin, S.D. & Springer, T.A. (1987). Purified intracellular adhesion molecule-1 (ICAM-1) is a ligand for lymphocyte function-associated antigen (LFA-1). *Cell*, **51**, 813–9.

Marr, D. (1969). A theory of cerebellar cortex. *Journal of Physiology*, **202**, 437–70.

Martini, R. & Schachner, M. (1988). Immunoelectronmicroscopic localization of neural cell adhesion molecules (L1, N-CAM and myelin-associated glycoprotein) in regenerating adult mouse sciatic nerve. *Journal of Cell Biology*, **106**, 1735–44.

Marx, J.L. (1986). Nerve growth factor acts in brain. *Science*, **232**, 1341–2.

Massoulié, J. & Bon, S. (1982). The molecular forms of cholinesterase in vertebrates. *Annual Review of Neuroscience*, **5**, 57–106.

Matthews, M.R., Cowan, W.M. & Powell, T.P.S. (1960). Transneuronal cell degeneration in the lateral geniculate nucleus of the macaque monkey. *Journal of Physiology*, **94**, 145–69.

McConnell, S.K. (1989). The determination of neuronal fate in the cerebral cortex. *Trends in Neurosciences*, **12**, 342–9.

McQuarrie, I.G. (1978). The effect of a conditioning lesion on the regeneration of motor axons. *Brain Research*, **152**, 597–602.

McQuarrie, I.G., Grafstein, B., Dreyfus, B.C.F. & Gershon, M.B. (1978). Regeneration of adrenergic axons in rat sciatic nerve: effect of a conditioning lesion. *Brain Research*, **141**, 21–34.

Menesini-Chen, M.G., Chen, J.S. & Levi-Montalcini, R. (1978). Sympathetic nerve fibre ingrowth in the CNS of neonatal rodent upon intracerebral NGF injections. *Archives Italiennes de Biologie*, **116**, 53–84.

Merlie, J.P. & Sanes, J.R. (1985). Concentration of acetylcholine receptor mRNA in synaptic regions of adult muscle fibres. *Nature*, **317**, 66–8.

Merzenich, M.M., Recanzone, G., Jenkins, W.M., Allan, T.T. & Nudo, R.J. (1988). Cortical Representational Plasticity. In *Neurobiology of Neocortex* (eds. P. Rakic & W. Singer), pp. 41–67. New York, John Wiley & Son Ltd.

Metzler, J. & Marks, P.J. (1979). Functional changes in cat somatic sensorimotor cortex during short term reversible epidural blocks. *Brain Research*, **177**, 379–83.

Meyer, R.L. (1980). Mapping the normal and regenerating retinotectal projection of goldfish with autoradiographic methods. *Journal of Comparative Neurology*, **189**, 273–89.

(1982). Tetrodotoxin blocks the formation of ocular dominance columns in goldfish. *Science*, **218**, 589–91.

(1984). Target selection by surgically misdirected optic fibres in the tectum of the goldfish. *Journal of Neuroscience*, **4**, 234–50.

(1987). Tests for relabelling the goldfish tectum by optic fibres. *Developmental Biology Research*, **31**, 312–8.

Milburn, A. (1973). The early development of muscle spindles in the rat. *Journal of Cell Science*, **12**, 175–95.

Miledi, R. & Slater, C.R. (1970). On the degeneration of rat neuromuscular junctions after nerve section. *Journal of Physiology*, **207**, 507–28.

Miledi, R. & Uchitel, O.D. (1981). Induction of action potentials in frog slow muscle fibres paralysed by alpha bungarotoxin. *Proceedings of the Royal Society of London*, **B213**, 243–8.

Miller, F.D., Tetzlaff, W., Bisby, M.A., Fawcett, J.W. & Milner, R.J. (1989). Rapid induction of the major embryonic α-tubulin mRNA, Tα1, during nerve regeneration in adult rats. *Journal of Neuroscience*, **9**, 1452–63.

Miller, J.B. & Stockdale, F.E. (1986). Developmental regulation of the multiple myogenic cell lineages of the avian embryo. *Journal of Cell Biology*, **103**, 2197–208.

(1987). What muscle cells know that nerves don't tell them. *Trends in Neurosciences*, **10**, 325–9.

Miner, N. (1956). Integumental specification of sensory fibres in the development of cutaneous local sign. *Journal of Comparative Neurology*, **105**, 161–71.

Mishima, M., Takai, T., Imoto, K., Noda, M. & Takahashi, T. (1986). Molecular distinction between fetal and adult forms of muscle acetylcholine receptor. *Nature*, **231**, 406–11.

Mitchison, T. & Kirschner, M. (1988). Cytoskeletal dynamics and nerve growth. *Neuron*, **1**, 761–72.

Monard, D. (1988). Cell-derived proteases and protease inhibitors as regulators of neurite outgrowth. *Trends in Neurosciences*, **11**, 541–4.

Montarolo, P.G., Goelet, P., Castelluci, V.F., Morgan, J., Kandel, E.R. & Schacher, S. (1986). A critical period for macromolecular synthesis in long-term heterosynaptic facilitation in *Aplysia*. *Science*, **234**, 1249–54.

Montell, D.J. & Goodman, C.S. (1988). *Drosophila* substrate adhesion molecule:

sequence of laminin B1 chain reveals domains of homology with mouse. *Cell*, **53**, 463–73.

Morest, D.K. (1969). The growth of dendrites in the mammalian brain. *Zeitschrift für Anatomie und Entwicklungsgeschichte*, **128**, 290–317.

Morris, R.G., Anderson, B., Lynch, G.S. & Baudry, M. (1986). Selective impairment of learning and blockade of long-term potentiation by an N-methyl-D-aspartate receptor antagonist, AP5. *Nature*, **319**, 774–6.

Muller, D., Joly, M. & Lynch, G. (1988). Contributions of quisqualate and NMDA receptors to the induction and expression of LTP. *Science*, **242**, 1694–7.

Murphey, R.K. (1985). Competition and chemoaffinity in insect sensory systems. *Trends in Neurosciences*, **8**, 120–5.

Murray, J.G. & Thompson, J.W. (1957). The occurrence and function of collateral sprouting in the sympathetic nervous system of the cat. *Journal of Physiology*, **135**, 133–62.

Murray, M.A. & Robbins, N. (1982*a*). Cell proliferation in denervated muscle: time course, distribution and relation to disease. *Neuroscience*, **7**, 1817–22.

(1982*b*). Cell proliferation in denervated muscle: identity and origin of dividing cells. *Neuroscience*, **7**, 1823–33.

Myers, P.Z., Eisen, J.S. & Westerfield, M. (1986). Development and axonal outgrowth of identified motor neurons in the Zebra fish. *Journal of Neuroscience*, **6**, 2278–89.

Nelson, R.B., Linden, D.J., Hyman, C., Pfenninger, K.H. & Routtenberg, A. (1989). The two major phosphoproteins in growth cones are probably identical to two protein kinase C substrates correlated with persistence of long-term potentiation. *Journal of Neuroscience*, **9**, 381–9.

Neugebauer, K.M., Tomaselli, K.J., Lilien, J. & Reichardt, L.F. (1988). N-cadherin, NCAM and integrins promote retinal neurite outgrowth on astrocytes in vitro. *Journal of Cell Biology*, **107**, 1177–87.

New, H.V. & Mudge, A.W. (1986). Calcitonin gene-related peptide regulates muscle acetylcholine receptor synthesis. *Nature*, **323**, 809–11.

Nilssen, O.G., Clarke, D.J., Brundin, P. & Björklund, A. (1988). Comparison of growth and reinnervation properties of cholinergic neurons from different brain regions grafted to the hippocampus. *Journal of Comparative Neurology*, **268**, 204–22.

Nishi, R. & Berg, D.K. (1981). Two components from eye tissue that differentially stimulate the growth and development of ciliary ganglion neurons in cell culture. *Journal of Neuroscience*, **1**, 505–13.

Nixon, R.A. (1987). The axonal transport of cytoskeletal proteins: a reappraisal. In *Axonal Transport* (ed. R.S. Smith & M.A. Bisby), pp. 175–200. New York, Alan R. Liss.

Njå, A. & Purves, D. (1977*a*). Specific innervation of guinea pig superior cervical ganglion cells by pre ganglionic fibres arising from different levels of the spinal cord. *Journal of Physiology*, **264**, 565–83.

(1977*b*). Reinnervation of guinea pig superior cervical ganglion cells by preganglionic fibres arising from different levels of the spinal cord. *Journal of Physiology*, **272**, 633–51.

(1978). The effects of nerve growth factor and its antiserum on synapses in the superior cervical ganglion of the guinea pig. *Journal of Physiology*, **277**, 53–75.

Noakes, P.G. & Bennett, M.R. (1987). Growth of axons into developing muscles of the chick forelimb is preceded by cells that stain with Schwann cell antibodies.

Journal of Comparative Neurology, **259**, 330–47.

Noakes, P.G., Bennett, M.R. & Stratford, J. (1988). Migration of Schwann cells and axons into developing chick forelimb muscles following removal of either the neural tube or the neural crest. *Journal of Comparative Neurology*, **277**, 214–33.

Nobin, A., Baumgarten, H.G., Björklund, A., Lachenmayer, L. & Stenevi, U. (1973). Axonal degeneration and regeneration of the bulbospinal indolamine neurons after 5,6 dihydroxytryptamine treatment. *Brain Research*, **56**, 1–24.

Nottebohm, F. (1970). Ontogeny of bird song. *Science*, **167**, 950–6.

Nurcombe, V. & Bennett, M.R. (1981). Embryonic chick retinal ganglion cells identified 'in vitro'. Their survival is dependent on a factor from the optic tectum. *Experimental Brain Research*, **44**, 244–58.

O'Brien, R.A.D., Ostberg, A.J.C. & Vrbova, G. (1978). Observations on the elimination of polyneuronal innervation in developing mammalian skeletal muscle. *Journal of Physiology*, **282**, 571–82.

    (1980). The effect of acetylcholine on the function and structure of the developing mammalian neuromuscular junction. *Neuroscience*, **5**, 1367–79.

O'Keefe, J. (1976). Place units in the hippocampus of the freely-moving rat. *Experimental Neurology*, **51**, 78–109.

O'Keefe, J. & Dostrovsky, J. (1971). The hippocampus as a spatial map. Preliminary evidence from unit activity in the freely-moving rat. *Brain Research*, **34**, 171–5.

O'Leary, D.D.M., Fawcett, J.W. & Cowan, W.M. (1986). Topographic targeting errors in the retino-collicular projection and their elimination by selective ganglion cell death. *Journal of Neuroscience*, **6**, 3692–705.

O'Leary, D.D.M., Stanfield, B.B. & Cowan, W.M. (1981). Evidence that the early postnatal restriction of the cells of origin of the callosal projection is due to the elimination of axon collaterals rather than to the death of neurons. *Developmental Brain Research*, **1**, 607–17.

O'Leary, D.D.M. & Terashima, T. (1988). Cortical axons branch to multiple subcortical targets by interstitial axon budding: implications for target recognition and waiting periods. *Neuron*, **1**, 901–10.

Ohsugi, K. & Ide, H. (1986). Position specific binding of a monoclonal antibody in chick limb buds. *Developmental Biology*, **117**, 676–9.

Okada, N. & Oppenheim, R.W. (1984). Cell death of motor neurons in the chick embryo spinal cord IX. The loss of motor neurons following removal of afferent input. *Journal of Neuroscience*, **4**, 1639–52.

Olton, D.S., Walker, J.A. & Gage, F.H. (1978). Hippocampal connections in spatial discrimination. *Brain Research*, **139**, 295–308.

Oppenheim, R.W. (1989). The neurotrophic theory and naturally occurring motor neuron death. *Trends in Neurosciences*, **12**, 252–4.

Oppenheim, R.W., Haverkamp, L.J., Prevette, D., McManaman, J.L. & Appel, S.H. (1988). Reduction of naturally occurring motor neuron death in vivo by a target-derived neurotrophic factor. *Science*, **240**, 919–22.

Oppenheim, R.W., Maderdrut, J.L. & Wells, D.J. (1982). Reduction of naturally occurring cell death in the thoraco lumbar preganglionic cell column of the chick embryo by nerve growth factor and hemicholinium 3. *Developmental Brain Research*, **3**, 134–9.

Oppenheim, R.W. & Nunez, R. (1982). Electrical stimulation of hind limb increases neuronal cell death in chick embryo. *Nature*, **295**, 57–9.

Ostberg, A.J., Raisman, G., Field, P.M., Iversen, L.L. & Zigmond, R.E. (1976). A quantitative comparison of the formation of synapses in the rat superior cervical ganglion by its own and by foreign nerve fibres. *Brain Research*, **107**, 445–70.

Palka, J. (1986). Neurogenesis and axonal pathfinding in invertebrates. *Trends in Neurosciences*, **9**, 482–5.

Pamphlett, R. (1988). Axonal sprouting after botulinum toxin does not elicit a histological axon reaction. *Journal of Neurological Science*, **87**, 175–85.

Panayatou, G., End, P., Aumailley, M., Timpl, R. & Engel, J. (1989). Domains of laminin with growth factor activity. *Cell*, **56**, 93–101.

Patel, N.H., Snow, P.M. & Goodman, C.S. (1987). Characterisation and cloning of fasciclin III: a glycoprotein expressed on a subset of neurons and axon pathways in *Drosophila*. *Cell*, **48**, 975–88.

Patterson, P.H. (1988). On the importance of being inhibited, or saying no to growth cones. *Neuron*, **1**, 263–7.

Patterson, P.H. & Chun, L.L.Y. (1977). The induction of acetylcholine synthesis in primary cultures of dissociated rat sympathetic neurons. *Developmental Biology*, **56**, 263–80.

Patterson, P.H., Potter, D.D. & Furshpan, E.J. (1978). The chemical differentiation of nerve cells. *Scientific American*, **239**, 38–47.

Paulsson, M., Deutzmonn, R., Timpl, R., Dalzoppo, D., Odermatt, E. & Engel, J. (1985). Evidence for coiled-coil alpha-helical regions in the long arm of laminin. *EMBO Journal*, **4**, 309–15.

Peng, H.B. & Cheng, P.-.C. (1982). Formation of postsynaptic specialisations induced by latex beads in cultured muscle cells. *Journal of Neuroscience*, **2**, 1760–74.

Perry, V.H. & Gordon, S. (1988). Macrophages and microglia in the nervous system. *Trends in Neurosciences*, **11**, 273–7.

Pette, D. & Staron, R.S. (1988). Molecular basis of the phenotypic characteristics of mammalian muscle fibres. *Ciba Foundation Symposium*, **138**, 22–34.

Pettigrew, J., Olson, C. & Barlow, H.B. (1973). Kitten visual cortex: short-term, stimulus-induced changes in connectivity. *Science*, **180**, 1202–3.

Pettigrew, J.D. (1974). The effect of visual experience on the development of stimulus specificity by kitten cortical neurons. *Journal of Physiology*, **237**, 49–74.

Pfenninger, K.H. (1986). Of nerve growth cones, leukocytes and memory : second messenger systems and growth regulated proteins. *Trends in Neurosciences*, **9**, 562–5.

Pitman, R.M. (1975). The ionic dependence of action potentials induced by colchicine in an insect motor neuron cell body. *Journal of Physiology*, **247**, 511–20.

Pittman, R.H. & Oppenheim, R.W. (1978). Neuromuscular blockade increases motor neuron survival during normal cell death in chick embryo. *Nature*, **271**, 364–6.

Pockett, S. & Slack, J.R. (1983). Ability of motor neurons to regulate quantal release and terminal growth after reduction in motor unit size. *Brain Research*, **258**, 296–8.

Price, J. (1987). Retroviruses and the study of cell lineage. *Development*, **101**, 409–19.

Purves, D. (1975). Functional and structural changes in mammalian sympathetic neurons following colchicine application to postganglionic nerves. *Journal of Physiology*, **259**, 159–75.

(1976). Competitive and non-competitive reinnervation of mammalian sympathetic neurons by native and foreign fibres. *Journal of Physiology*, **261**, 453–75.

(1988). *Body and Brain*. Harvard, Harvard University Press.

Purves, D. & Hadley, R.D. (1985). Changes in the dendritic branching of adult mammalian neurones revealed by repeated imaging in vitro. *Nature*, **315**, 404–6.

Purves, D. & Lichtman, J.W. (1980). Elimination of synapses in the developing nervous system. *Science*, **210**, 153–7.

Purves, D., Rubin, E., Snider, W.D. & Lichtman, J. (1986). Relation of animal size to convergence, divergence and neuronal number in peripheral sympathetic pathways. *Journal of Neuroscience*, **6**, 158–63.

Purves, D., Snider, W.D. & Voyvodic, J.T. (1988). Trophic regulation of nerve cell morphology and innervation in the autonomic nervous system. *Nature*, **336**, 123–8.

Purves, D. & Thompson, W. (1979). The effects of post ganglionic axotomy on selective sympathetic connections in the superior cervical ganglion of the guinea pig. *Journal of Physiology*, **297**, 95–110.

Purves, D., Thompson, W. & Yip, J.W. (1981). Reinnervation of ganglia transplanted to the neck from different levels of the guinea pig sympathetic chain. *Journal of Physiology*, **313**, 49–63.

Radeke, M.J., Misko, T.P., Hsu, C., Herzenberg, L.A. & Shooter, E.M. (1987). Gene transfer and molecular cloning of the rat nerve growth factor receptor: a new class of receptors. *Nature*, **325**, 593–7.

Raff, M.C. (1989). Glial cell diversification in the rat optic nerve. *Science*, **243**, 1450–5.

Raisman, G. & Field, P.M. (1973). A quantitative investigation of the development of collateral reinnervation after partial deafferentation of septal nuclei. *Brain Research*, **50**, 241–64.

Rakic, P. (1971). Neuron–glia relationship during granule cell migration in developing cerebellar cortex. *Journal of Comparative Neurology*, **141**, 283–312.

(1972). Mode of cell migration to the superficial layers of fetal monkey neocortex. *Journal of Comparative Neurology*, **145**, 61–84.

(1975). Role of cell interaction in development of dendritic patterns. *Advances in Neurology*, **12**, 117–34.

(1977a). Genesis of the dorsal lateral geniculate nucleus in the rhesus monkey. *Journal of Comparative Neurology*, **176**, 23–52.

(1977b). Prenatal development of the visual system in Rhesus monkey. *Philosophical Transactions of the Royal Society B*, **278**, 245–260.

(1981). Development of visual centres in the primate brain depends on binocular competition before birth. *Science*, **214**, 928–31.

(1986). Mechanisms of ocular dominance segregation in the lateral geniculate nucleus: competitive elimination hypothesis. *Trends in Neurosciences*, **9**, 11–15.

(1988). Specification of cerebral cortical areas. *Science*, **241**, 170–6.

Raper, J.A., Bastiani, M. & Goodman, C.S. (1983). Pathfinding by neuronal growth cones in grasshopper embryos. II. Selective fasciculation with specific axonal pathways. *Journal of Neuroscience*, **3**, 31–41.

Ratner, N., Hong, D., Lieberman, M.A., Bunge, R.B. & Glaser, L. (1988). The neuronal cell-surface molecule mitogenic for Schwann cells is a heparin-binding proteoglycan. *Proceedings of the National Academy of Science U.S.A.*, **85**, 6992–6.

Rauschecker, J.P. & Singer, W. (1981). The effects of early visual experience on the cat's visual cortex and their possible explanation by Hebb synapses. *Journal of Physiology*, **310**, 215–39.

Ready, D.F. (1989). A multifaceted approach to neural development. *Trends in Neurosciences*, **12**, 102–10.

Redfern, P.A. (1970). Neuromuscular transmission in newborn rats. *Journal of Physiology*, **209**, 701–9.

Reh, T.A. & Constantine-Paton, M. (1985). Eye specific segregation requires neural activity in three-eyed *R. pipiens*. *Journal of Neuroscience*, **5**, 1132–43.

Ribchester, R.R. (1988). Activity-dependent and -independent synaptic interactions during reinnervation of partially denervated rat muscle. *Journal of Physiology*, **401**, 53–75.

Ribchester, R.R. & Taxt, T. (1983). Motor unit size and synaptic competition in rat lumbrical muscles reinnervated by active and inactive motor axons. *Journal of Physiology*, **344**, 89–111.

Rich, M.M. & Lichtman, J.W. (1989). In vivo visualization of pre- and post-synaptic changes during synapse elimination in reinnervated mouse muscle. *Journal of Neuroscience*, **9**, 1781–1805.

Richardson, P.M., McGuiness, U.M. & Aguayo, A.J. (1980). Axons from CNS neurones regenerate into PNS grafts. *Nature*, **284**, 264–5.

Richman, D.P., Steward, R.M., Hutchinson, H.W. & Caviness, V.S. (1975). Mechanical model of brain convolutional development. *Science*, **189**, 18–21.

Ridge, R.M.A.P. & Betz, W.J. (1984). The effect of selective chronic stimulation on motor unit size in developing rat muscle. *Journal of Neuroscience*, **4**, 2614–20.

Ridley, A.J., Davis, J.B., Stroobant, P. & Land, H. (1989). Transforming Growth Factors $\beta1$ and $\beta2$ are mitogens for rat Schwann cells. *Journal of Cell Biology*, **109**, 3419–24.

Riley, D.A. (1976). Multiple axon branches innervating single endplates of kitten soleus myofibres. *Brain Research*, **110**, 158–61.

(1977). Spontaneous elimination of nerve terminals from the endplates of developing skeletal myofibres. *Brain Research*, **134**, 279–85.

(1981). Ultrastructural evidence for axon retraction during the spontaneous elimination of polyneuronal innervation of the rat soleus muscle. *Journal of Neurocytology*, **10**, 425–40.

Rodriguez-Boulan, E. & Nelson, W.J. (1989). Morphogenesis of the epithelial cell phenotype. *Science*, **245**, 718–25.

Rosenthal, J.L. & Taraskevich, S.P. (1977). Reduction in multiaxonal innervation of the neuromuscular junction of the rat during development. *Journal of Physiology*, **270**, 299–310.

Ross, J.J., Duxson, M.J. & Harris, A.J. (1987). Neural determination of muscle fibre number in embryonic rat lumbrical muscles. *Development*, **100**, 395–410.

Rotshenker, S. (1979). Synapse formation in intact innervated cutaneous pectoris muscles of the frog following denervation of the opposite muscle. *Journal of Physiology*, **292**, 535–47.

Rubin, E. (1985). Development of the rat superior cervical ganglion: initial stages of synapse formation. *Journal of Neuroscience*, **5**, 697–704.

Rutishauser, U., Grumet, M. & Edelman, G.M. (1983). Neural cell adhesion molecule mediates initial interactions between spinal cord neurons and muscle cells in culture. *Journal of Cell Biology*, **97**, 145–52.

Rutishauser, U. & Jessell, T.M. (1988). Cell adhesion molecules in vertebrate neural development. *Physiological Reviews*, **68**, 819–57.

Saade, N.E., Banna, N.R., Khoury, A., Jabbur, S.J. & Wall, P.D. (1982). Cutaneous receptive field alterations induced by 4 aminopyridine. *Brain Research*, **232**, 177–80.

Salmons, S. & Sreter, F.A. (1976). Significance of impulse activity in the transformation of skeletal muscle types. *Nature*, **263**, 30–4.

Sanes, D.H. & Constantine Paton, M. (1983). Altered activity patterns during development reduce neural tuning. *Science*, **221**, 1183–4.

Sanes, J.R. (1989a). Analysing cell lineage with a recombinant retrovirus. *Trends in Neurosciences*, **12**, 21–8.

(1989b). Extracellular matrix molecules that influence neural development. *Annual Review of Neuroscience*, **12**, 491–516.

Sanes, J.R., Marshall, L.M. & McMahan, U.J. (1978). Reinnervation of muscle fibre basal lamina after removal of myofibres. *Journal of Cell Biology*, **78**, 176–98.

Sargent, P.B. (1989). What distinguishes axons from dendrites? Neurons know more than we do. *Trends in Neurosciences*, **12**, 203–5.

Saxen, L. (1980). Neural induction: past present and future. *Current Topics in Developmental Biology*, **15**, 409–18.

Sayers, H. & Tonge, D.A. (1982). Differences between foreign and original innervation of skeletal muscle in the frog. *Journal of Physiology*, **330**, 57–68.

Schlessinger, A.R., Cowan, W.M. & Gottlieb, D.I. (1975). An autoradiographic study of the time of origin and the pattern of granule cell migration in the dentate gyrus of the rat. *Journal of Comparative Neurology*, **159**, 149–76.

Schmidt, H. & Stefani, E. (1977). Action potentials in slow muscle fibres of the frog during regeneration of motor nerves. *Journal of Physiology*, **270**, 507–17.

Schmidt, J.T. (1984). Natural history of optic arbors on the tectum of fish and frog. *Trends in Neurosciences*, **7**, 358–60.

Scholes, J.H. (1979). Nerve fibre topography in the retinal projection to the tectum. *Nature*, **278**, 620–4.

Schotzinger, R.J. & Landis, S.C. (1988). Cholinergic phenotype developed by noradrenergic sympathetic neurons after innervation of a novel cholinergic target in vivo. *Nature*, **335**, 637–9.

Schuetze, S.M. & Role, L.W. (1987). Developmental regulation of the nicotinic acetylcholine receptor. *Annual Review of Neuroscience*, **10**, 403–57.

Schwab, M.E. & Caroni, P. (1988). Oligodendrocytes and CNS myelin are nonpermissive substrates for neurite growth and fibroblast spreading in vitro. *Journal of Neuroscience*, **8**, 2381–93.

Schwarz, J.P., Pearson, J. & Johnson, E.M. (1982). Effects of exposure to anti NGF on sensory neurons of adult rats and guinea pigs. *Brain Research*, **244**, 378–81.

Scott, S.A. (1975). Persistence of foreign innervation on reinnervated goldfish extraocular muscles. *Science*, **189**, 644–6.

(1982). The development of the segmental pattern of skin sensory innervation in embryonic chick hind limb. *Journal of Physiology*, **330**, 203–20.

(1987). The development of skin sensory innervation patterns. *Trends in Neurosciences*, **10**, 468–73.

Scott, S.A., Cooper, E. & Diamond, J. (1981). Merkel cells as targets of the mechanosensory nerves in salamander skin. *Proceedings of the Royal Society of London*, **B211**, 455–70.

Selzer, Z. & Devor, M. (1984). Effect of nerve section on the spinal distribution of neighbouring nerves. *Brain Research*, **306**, 31–7.

Shankland, M. (1987). Position-dependent cell interactions and commitments in the formation of the leech nervous system. *Current Topics in Developmental Biology*, **21**, 31–63.

Sharpe, C.R., Fritz, A. & DeRobertis, E.M. (1987). A homeobox-containing marker of posterior neural differentiation shows the importance of predetermination in neural induction. *Cell*, **50**, 749–58.

Shieh, P. (1951). The neoformation of cells of preganglionic type in the cervical spinal cord of the chick embryo following its transplantation to the thoracic level. *Journal of Experimental Zoology*, **117**, 354–95.

Silver, J., Lorenz, S.E., Wahlsten, D. & Coughlin, J. (1982). Axonal guidance during development of the great cerebral commissures: descriptive and experimental studies, *in vivo*, on the role of preformed pathways. *Journal of Comparative Neurology*, **210**, 10–29.

Silver, J. & Sapiro, J. (1981). Axonal guidance during development of the optic nerve: the role of pigmented epithelia and other extrinsic factors. *Journal of Comparative Neurology*, **202**, 521–38.

Simpson, S.A. & Young, J.Z. (1945). Regeneration of fibre diameter after cross unions of visceral and somatic nerves. *Journal of Anatomy*, **79**, 48–65.

Singer, M. (1974). Neurotrophic control of limb regeneration in the newt. *Annals of the New York Academy of Sciences*, **228**, 308–22.

Singer, M., Norlander, R.H. & Egar, M. (1979). Axonal guidance during embryogenesis and regeneration in the spinal cord of the newt: the blueprint hypothesis of neuronal pathway patterning. *Journal of Comparative Neurology*, **185**, 1–22.

Singer, P.A. & Mehler, S. (1980). ^{2}-deoxy-^{14}C-glucose uptake in rat hypoglossal nucleus after nerve transection. *Experimental Neurology*, **69**, 617–26.

Skene, J.H.P. (1984). Growth-associated proteins and the curious dichotomies of nerve regeneration. *Cell*, **37**, 697–700.

(1989). Axonal growth-associated proteins. *Annual Review of Neuroscience*, **12**, 127–56.

Skoff, R.D. & Hamburger, V. (1974). Fine structure of dendritic and axonal growth cones in embryonic chick spinal cord. *Journal of Comparative Neurology*, **153**, 107–48.

Slack, J.R. & Hopkins, W.G. (1982). Neuromuscular transmission at terminals of sprouted mammalian motor neurons. *Brain Research*, **237**, 121–35.

Slack, J.R. & Pockett, S. (1981). Terminal sprouting is a local response to a local stimulus. *Brain Research*, **217**, 368–74.

Smith, G.M., Miller, R.H. & Silver, J. (1986). Changing role of forebrain astrocytes during development, regenerative failure and induced regeneration upon transplantation using mouse callosum. *Journal of Comparative Neurology*, **251**, 23–43.

Smith, J.C. (1989). Mesoderm induction and mesoderm-inducing factors in early amphibian development. *Development*, **105**, 665–7.

Smith, M.A., Yao, Y.M.M., Reist, N.E., Magill, C., Wallace, B.G. & McMahan, U.J. (1987). Identification of agrin in electric organ extracts and localization of agrin-like molecules in muscle and central nervous system. *Journal of Experimental Biology*, **132**, 223–30.

Smith, R.G., Vaca, K., McManaman, J. & Appel, S.H. (1986). Selective effects of skeletal muscle extract fractions in motor neuron development in vitro. *Journal of Neuroscience*, **6**, 439–47.

Smolen, A.J. (1981). Postnatal development of ganglionic neurons in the absence of preganglionic input: morphological observations on synaptic formation. *Developmental Brain Research*, **1**, 49–58.

Soha, J.M., Yo, C. & Van Essen, D.C. (1987). Synapse elimination by fibre type and maturational state in rabbit soleus muscle. *Developmental Biology*, **123**, 136–44.

Speidel, C.C. (1942). Studies of living nerves. VII. Growth adjustments of cutaneous terminal arborizations. *Journal of Comparative Neurology*, **76**, 57–69.

Spemann, H. (1938). *Embryonic Development and Induction*. New House, Yale University Press.

Sperry, R.W. (1943). Effects of 180 degree rotation of the retinal field on visuo motor coordination. *Journal of Experimental Zoology*, **92**, 263–79.

(1963). Chemoaffinity in the orderly growth of nerve fibre patterns and connections. *Proceedings of the National Academy of Science U.S.A.*, **50**, 703–10.

Spitzer, N. (1981). Development of membrane properties in vertebrates. *Trends in Neurosciences*, **4**, 19–22.

Sretavan, D.W. & Shatz, C.J. (1986). Prenatal development of retinal ganglion cell axons: segregation into eye-specific layers within the cat's lateral geniculate nucleus. *Journal of Neuroscience*, **6**, 234–51.

Stanfield, B.B., O'Leary, D.D.M. & Fricks, C. (1982). Selective collateral elimination in early postnatal development restricts cortical distribution of rat pyramidal tract neurones. *Nature*, **298**, 371–3.

Stent, G.S. & Weisblat, D.A. (1981). Cell lineage in the development of the leech nervous system. *Trends in Neurosciences*, **4**, 251–55.

Stern, C.D., Norris, W.E., Bronner Fraser, M., Carlson, G.J., Faissner, A., Keynes, R.J. & Schachner, M. (1989). J1/tenascin-related molecules are not responsible for the segmented pattern of neural crest cells or motor axons in the chick embryo. *Development*, **107**, 309–19.

Sternberg, P.W. (1988). Control of cell fates within equivalence groups in *C. elegans*. *Trends in Neurosciences*, **11**, 259–64.

Stockel, K., Paravicini, U. & Thoenen, H. (1974). Specificity of the retrograde axonal transport of nerve growth factor. *Brain Research*, **76**, 413–21.

Straznicky, C., Gaze, R.M. & Keating, M.J. (1981). The development of the retinotectal projections from compound eyes in *Xenopus*. *Journal of Embryology and Experimental Morphology*, **62**, 13–35.

Stryker, M.P. & Harris, W.A. (1986). Binocular impulse traffic blockade prevents the formation of ocular dominance columns in cat visual cortex. *Journal of Neuroscience*, **6**, 2117–33.

Stryker, M.P. & Sherk, H. (1975). Modification of cortical orientation selectivity in the cat by restricted visual experience : a re-examination. *Science*, **190**, 904–5.

Sulston, J.E. & Horvitz, H.R. (1977). Post embryonic cell lineages of the nematode *Caenorhabditis elegans*. *Developmental Biology*, **56**, 110–56.

Sulston, J.E. & White, J. (1980). Regulation and cell autonomy during postembryonic development of *Caenorhabditis elegans*. *Developmental Biology*, **78**, 577–97.

Summerbell, D. & Stirling, R.V. (1981). The innervation of dorso ventrally reversed chick wings: evidence that motor axons do not actively seek out their appropriate targets. *Journal of Embryology and Experimental Morphology*, **61**, 233–47.

Sunderland, S. (1978). *Nerves and Nerve Injuries.* 2nd edition. London, Churchill Livingston.

Suzue, T., Imrick, J. & Patterson, P.H. (1988). Monoclonal antibodies that define rostro-caudal position in the mammalian nervous system. *Society Neuroscience Abstracts,* **14**, 596.

Swanson, G.J. & Lewis, J. (1986). Sensory nerve routes in chick wing buds deprived of motor innervation. *Journal of Embryology and Experimental Morphology,* **95**, 37–52.

Sweadner, K.J. (1983). Post-translational modification and evoked release of two large surface proteins of sympathetic neurons. *Journal of Neuroscience,* **3**, 2504–17.

Swindale, N.V. (1981). Absence of ocular dominance patches in dark reared cats. *Nature,* **290**, 332–3.

Takeichi, M. (1988). The cadherins: cell–cell adhesion molecules controlling animal morphogenesis. *Development,* **102**, 639–55.

Tanaka, H. & Landmesser, L.T. (1986*a*). Interspecies selective motor neuron projection patterns in chick–quail chimeras. *Journal of Neuroscience,* **6**, 2880–8.

Tanaka, H. & Landmesser, L.M. (1986*b*). Cell death of lumbosacral motor neurons in chick, quail and chick–quail chimera embryos. *Journal of Neuroscience,* **6**, 2889–99.

Teller, D.Y. & Movshon, J.A. (1986). Visual development. *Vision Research,* **26**, 1483–1506.

Tessier-Lavigne, M., Placzek, M., Lumsden, A.G.S., Dodd, J. & Jessell, T.M. (1988). Chemotropic guidance of developing axons in the mammalian central nervous system. *Nature,* **336**, 775–8.

Tetzlaff, W. & Bisby, M.A. (1988). Changes in gene expression following axotomy are similar in rubrospinal (CNS) and facial (PNS) neurons. *Society Neuroscience Abstracts,* **14**, 323.14.

Tetzlaff, W. & Bisby, M.A. (1989). Neurofilament elongation into regenerating facial nerve axons. *Neuroscience,* **29**, 659–66.

Tetzlaff, W., Bisby, M.A. & Kreutzberg, G.W. (1988). Changes in cytoskeletal proteins in the rat facial nucleus following axotomy. *Journal of Neuroscience,* **8**, 3181–9.

Thanos, S., Bonhoeffer, F. & Rutishauser, U. (1984). Fibre–fibre interaction and tectal cues influence the development of the chicken retino-tectal projection. *Proceedings of the National Academy of Science,* **81**, 1906–10.

Thoenen, H., Angeletti, P.V., Levi Montalcini, R. & Kettler, R. (1971). Selective induction by nerve growth factor of tyrosine hydroxylase and dopamine β hydroxylase in the rat superior cervical ganglia. *Proceedings of the National Academy of Science U.S.A.,* **68**, 1598–602.

Thoenen, H. & Barde, T.A. (1980). Physiology of Nerve Growth Factor. *Physiological Reviews,* **60**, 1284–335.

Thompson, W. (1983). Synapse elimination in neonatal rat muscles is sensitive to the pattern of use. *Nature,* **302**, 614–6.

Thompson, W., Kuffler, D.P. & Jansen, J.K.S. (1979). The effect of prolonged reversible block of nerve impulses on the elimination of polyneuronal innervation of new-born rat skeletal muscle fibres. *Neuroscience,* **4**, 271–81.

Thompson, W.J., Sutton, L.A. & Riley, D.A. (1984). Fibre type composition of single motor units during synapse elimination in neonatal rat soleus muscle. *Nature,* **309**, 709–11.

Tomaselli, K.J., Neugebauer, L.M., Bixby, J.L., Lilien, J. & Reichardt, L.F. (1988). N-Cadherin and integrins: two receptor systems that mediate neuronal process outgrowth on astrocyte surfaces. *Neuron*, **1**, 33–43.

Tomlinson, A. (1988). Cellular interactions in the developing *Drosophila* eye. *Development*, **104**, 183–93.

Tosney, K.W. & Landmesser, L. (1985). Growth cone morphology and trajectory in the lumbosacral region of the chick embryo. *Journal of Neuroscience*, **5**, 2345–58.

Tosney, K.W., Schroeter, S. & Pokrzywinski, J.A. (1988). Cell death delineates axon pathways in the hindlimb and does so independently of neurite outgrowth. *Developmental Biology*, **130**, 558–72.

Tosney, K.W., Watanabe, M., Landmesser, L. & Rutishauser, U. (1986). The distribution of N-CAM in the chick hindlimb during axon outgrowth and synaptogenesis. *Developmental Biology*, **114**, 468–81.

Toutant, M., Bourgeois, J.P., Toutant, J.P., Renaud, D., Le Douarin G., Changeux, J-P. (1980). Chronic stimulation of the spinal cord in developing chick embryo causes the differentiation of multiple clusters of acetylcholine receptors in the posterior latissimus dorsi muscle. *Developmental Biology*, **76**, 384–95.

Tracey, K.J., Lowry, S.F., Beutler, B., Cerami, A., Albert, J.D. & Shires, G.T. (1986). Cachectin/tumor necrosis factor mediates changes of skeletal muscle membrane potential. *Journal of Experimental Medicine*, **164**, 1368–73.

Trisler, G.D., Schneider, M.D. & Nirenberg, M. (1981). A topographic gradient of molecules in retina can be used to identify neuron position. *Proceedings of the National Academy of Science U.S.A*, **78**, 2145–9.

Trisler, D. & Collins, F. (1987). Corresponding spatial gradients of TOP molecules in the developing retina and optic tectum. *Science*, **237**, 1208–9.

Truman, J.W. (1984). Cell death in invertebrate nervous systems. *Annual Review of Neuroscience*, **7**, 171–88.

Truman, J.W. & Reiss, S.E. (1976). Dendritic reorganization of an identified motor neuron during metamorphosis of the tobacco hornworm moth. *Science*, **192**, 477–9.

Trussell, L.D. & Grinnell, A.D. (1985). The regulation of synaptic strength within motor units of the frog cutaneous pectoris muscle. *Journal of Neuroscience*, **5**, 243–54.

Tsukahara, N. (1981). Sprouting and the neuronal basis of learning. *Trends in Neurosciences*, **4**, 234–7.

Turner, D. & Cepko, C. (1987). Cell lineage in the rat retina: a common progenitor for neurons and glia persists late in development. *Nature*, **328**, 131–6.

Turner, J.E. & Glaze, K.A. (1977). Regenerative repair in the severed optic nerve of the newt (*Triturus viridescens*): effect of nerve growth factor. *Experimental Neurology*, **57**, 687–97.

Turner, J.E., Schwab, M.E. & Thoenen, M. (1982). NGF stimulates neurite outgrowth from goldfish retinal explants: the influence of a prior lesion. *Developmental Brain Research*, **4**, 59–86.

Usherwood, P.N.R. (1969). Glutamate sensitivity of denervated insect muscle fibres. *Nature*, **223**, 411–3.

Valverde, F. (1967). Apical dendritic spines of the visual cortex and light deprivation in the mouse. *Experimental Brain Research*, **3**, 337–53.

Van der Loos, H. & Woolsey, T.A. (1973). Somatosensory cortex: structural alterations following early injury to sense organs. *Science*, **179**, 395–8.

Vanselow, J., Thanos, S., Godement, P., Henke Fahle, S. & Bonhoeffer, F. (1989). Spatial arrangement of glia and ingrowing retinal axons in the chick optic tectum during development. *Developmental Brain Research*, **45**, 15–27.

Varon, S., Skaper, S.D. & Manthorpe, M. (1981). Trophic activities for dorsal root and sympathetic ganglionic neurons in media conditioned by Schwann and other peripheral cells. *Developmental Brain Research*, **1**, 73–87.

Von der Malsburg, C. & Singer, W. (1988). Principles of cortical network organization. In *Neurobiology of Neocortex* (ed. P. Rakic & W. Singer), pp. 69–99. Chichester, John Wiley & Sons.

Voyvodic, J. T. (1989a). Peripheral target regulation of dendritic geometry in the rat superior cervical ganglion. *Journal of Neuroscience*, **9**, 1997–2010.

(1989b). Target size regulates calibre and myelination of sympathetic axons. *Nature*, **342**, 430–3.

Vrbova, G. (1988). Reorganisation of nerve–muscle synapses during development. In *Growth and Plasticity of Neural Connections* (ed. W.R. Winlow & C.R.McCrohan), pp. 22–35. Manchester University Press.

Wall, P.D. & Devor, M. (1981). The effect of peripheral nerve injury on dorsal root potentials and on transmission of afferent segments into the spinal cord. *Brain Research*, **209**, 95–111.

Walter, J., Kern Veils, B., Huf, J., Stolze, B. & Bonhoeffer, F. (1987). Recognition of position-specific properties of tectal cell membranes by retinal axons in vitro. *Development*, **101**, 685–96.

Warner, A.E. (1985). Factors controlling the early development of the nervous system. In *Molecular Bases of Neural Development* (ed. G.M. Edelman, W.E. Gall & W.M. Cowan). New York, John Wiley & Sons.

Watson, W.E. (1974). Cellular responses to axotomy and to related procedures. *British Medical Bulletin*, **30**, 112–5.

Weinberg, C.B. & Hall, Z.W. (1979). Junctional form of acetylcholinesterase restored at nerve free endplates. *Developmental Biology*, **68**, 631–5.

Weinberg, H.J. & Spencer, P.S. (1978). The fate of Schwann cells isolated from axonal contact. *Journal of Neurocytology*, **7**, 555–69.

Weldon, P.R., Moody Corbett, F. & Cohen, M.W. (1981). Ultrastructure of sites of cholinesterase activity on Amphibian embryonic muscle cells cultured without nerve. *Developmental Biology*, **84**, 341–50.

Werner, J.K. (1973). Mixed intra- and extra-fusal muscle fibres produced by temporary denervation in newborn rats. *Journal of Comparative Neurology*, **150**, 279–302.

Westgaard, R.H. (1975). Influence of activity on the passive electrical properties of denervated soleus fibres in the rat. *Journal of Physiology*, **251**, 683–97.

Westgaard, R.H. & Lømo, T. (1988). Control of contractile properties within adaptive ranges by patterns of impulse activity in the rat. *Journal of Neuroscience*, **8**, 4415–26.

Whitelaw, V.A. & Cowan, J.D. (1981). Specificity and plasticity of retino-tectal connections: a computational model. *Journal of Neuroscience*, **1**, 1369–87.

Wiesel, T.N. (1982). Postnatal development of the visual cortex and the influence of the environment. *Nature*, **299**, 583–91.

Wiesel, T.N. & Hubel, D.H. (1974). Ordered arrangement of orientation columns in monkeys lacking visual experience. *Journal of Comparative Neurology*, **158**, 307–18.

Wigston, D.J. & Donahue, S.P. (1988). The location of cues promoting selective reinnervation of axolotl muscles. *Journal of Neuroscience*, **8**, 3451–8.

Wigston, D.J. & Sanes, J.R. (1982). Selective reinnervation of adult mammalian muscle by axons from different segmental levels. *Nature*, **299**, 464–7.

(1985). Selective reinnervation of intercostal muscle transplanted from different segmental levels to a common site. *Journal of Neuroscience*, **5**, 1208–21.

Wilkinson, D.G., Bhatt, S., Cook, M., Boncinelli, E. & Krumlauf, R. (1989). Segmental expression of Hox-2 homoeobox-containing genes in the developing mouse hindbrain. *Nature*, **341**, 405–9.

Williams, A.F. (1985). Immunoglobulin-related domains for cell surface recognition. *Nature*, **314**, 579–80.

Williams, R.F. & Rakic, P. (1988). Elimination of neurons from the Rhesus monkey's lateral geniculate nucleus during development. *Journal of Comparative Neurology*, **272**, 424–36.

Wilson, P. & Snow, R.J. (1987). Reorganisation of the receptive fields of spinocervical tract neurons following denervation of a single digit in the cat. *Journal of Neurophysiology*, **57**, 803–18.

Wilson, S., Tonge, D.A. & Holder, N. (1989). Homing behavior of regenerating axons in the amphibian limb. *Development*, **100**, 707–15.

Yamamori, T., Fukada, K., Aebersold, R., Korsching, S., Fann, M.J. & Patterson, P.H. (1989). The cholinergic neuronal differentiation factor from heart cells is identical to leukaemia inhibitory factor. *Science*, **246**, 1412–6.

Yip, H.K., Rich, K.M., Lampe, P.A. & Johnson, E.M. (1984). The effects of Nerve Growth Factor and its antiserum on the postnatal development and survival after injury of sensory neurons in rat dorsal root ganglia. *Journal of Neuroscience*, **4**, 2986–92.

Zalewski, A.A. (1969). Combined effects of testosterone and motor, sensory or gustatory nerve reinnervation on the regeneration of taste buds. *Experimental Neurology*, **24**, 285–97.

(1981). Regeneration of taste buds after reinnervation of a denervated tongue papilla by a nongustatory nerve. *Journal of Comparative Neurology*, **220**, 309–14.

Zelena, J. (1964). Development, degeneration and regeneration of receptor organs. *Progress in Brain Research*, **13**, 175–213.

Zigmond, R.E. & Bowers, C.W. (1981). Influence of nerve activity on the macromolecular content of neurons and their effector organs. *Annual Review of Physiology*, **43**, 673–87.

Zigmond, R.E., Schwarzschild, A. & Rittenhouse, A.R. (1989). Acute regulation of tyrosine hydroxylase by nerve activity and by neurotransmitters via phosphorylation. *Annual Review of Neuroscience*, **12**, 415–61.

Index